CW00411109

Watson's Clinical Nursing Pocketbook

For Elsevier:

Commissioning Editor: Ninette Premdas
Development Editor: Sheila Black
Project Manager: Gail Wright
Designer: Erik Bigland
Illustration Manager: Bruce Hogarth

Watson's Clinical Nursing Pocketbook

SECOND EDITION

Mike Walsh BA PhD PCE RGN DipN

Reader in Nursing Studies, University of Cumbria, Carlisle, UK

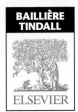

BAILLIÈRE
TINDALL

ELSEVIER

Edinburgh London New York Oxford Philadelphia St Louis Sydney Toronto 2008

BAILLIÈRE
TINDALL
ELSEVIER

© 2004 Elsevier Science Ltd
© 2008, Elsevier Limited. All rights reserved.

First edition 2004
Second edition 2008

ISBN 978-0-7020-2919-6

British Library Cataloguing in Publication Data
A catalogue record for this book is available from the British Library

Library of Congress Cataloging in Publication Data
A catalog record for this book is available from the Library of Congress

Notice
Knowledge and best practice in this field are constantly changing. As new
research and experience broaden our knowledge, changes in practice,
treatment and drug therapy may become necessary or appropriate.
Readers are advised to check the most current information provided (i)
on procedures featured or (ii) by the manufacturer of each product to be
administered, to verify the recommended dose or formula, the method
and duration of administration, and contraindications. It is the
responsibility of the practitioner, relying on their own experience and
knowledge of the patient, to make diagnoses, to determine dosages and
the best treatment for each individual patient, and to take all appropriate
safety precautions. To the fullest extent of the law, neither the Publisher
nor the Author assumes any liability for any injury and/or damage to
persons or property arising out or related to any use of the material
contained in this book.

The Publisher

Printed in China

Contents

Using this book   vii

1 The cardiovascular system   1

2 Caring for the patient with respiratory problems   17

3 Caring for the patient with a haematological
   disorder   35

4 Caring for the patient with a disorder of the
   gastrointestinal system   51

5 Caring for the patient with a disorder of the
   liver, biliary tract and exocrine pancreas   67

6 Caring for the patient with a disorder of the
   endocrine system   85

7 Caring for the patient with a disorder of the
   urinary system   107

8 Women's health   127

9 Caring for the patient with a disorder of the
   nervous system   143

Index   167

Using this book

This book has been designed for use during clinical practice, particularly at handover times, rather than for study at home in the evening or in college. It will allow you ready access to the key facts that you need for patient care during practice. Handover times at the start of a shift in hospital contain a great deal of information, and this book will help you to make rapid sense of the priorities for your patient over the shift ahead and beyond that to eventual discharge home. The book also incorporates care from the primary health perspective, so will be equally useful as a rapid read during community placements.

This rationale explains the structure of each chapter:

- a simple outline in diagrammatic form of the main anatomy of each body system
- a rapid read of the key elements of physiology
- a selection of the most common and serious conditions that you will encounter for that system.

Each condition contains a brief summary of the key facts you need to know about the disease itself (pathology). How the condition affects the patient is presented under the heading 'What to look out for', which summarizes key signs and symptoms. The 'Medical management' section explains what the doctors are attempting to do. It is important to understand the medical approach if nursing care is to be planned properly. Pharmacology is becoming increasingly important to nurses, hence the 'Pharmacology focus' section, which underlines the key elements in the pharmacological approach to treating the various conditions. Finally, and perhaps most importantly, there is an outline of the 'Nursing care priorities' required for adult patients with the condition.

At the end of each chapter, there are 'Ten top tips' to remind you of the most important aspects of caring for patients with disorders of that particular system.

This is not a comprehensive textbook. It is the clinical practice companion to *Watson's Clinical Nursing and Related Sciences*, 7th edition, and is designed to be used in conjunction with that book. It is cross-referenced throughout to the key sections in *Watson's* to enable you to follow up, later, on the patients you have seen during the day. Reading the appropriate section in *Watson's* subsequently will deepen and expand your understanding of the conditions that you have encountered during the day, their treatments, long-term management, and the implications they have for the whole lifestyle of the patient and family. The extra online resources that are available with *Watson's* will allow you to deepen your knowledge further with narrated PowerPoint lectures and case studies.

When reading *Watson's* after your shift, you can reflect upon the similarities and differences between your patient and the text. Patients rarely correspond exactly to the textbook situation, and sometimes there are very significant differences. Think about why such major discrepancies occur and what the implications are for nursing care. In this way, you will learn to move from a rapid read of the key facts contained in this book through the more in-depth analysis of *Watson's* and on to the essence of individualized nursing care: delivering care to meet the needs of the real and individual patient. These two books therefore complement each other and, used together in the way suggested above, should greatly facilitate your learning experience.

Mike Walsh
Carlisle 2007

1

The cardiovascular system

Anatomy at a glance   1
Physiology you need to know   1
Angina pectoris   3
Myocardial infarction   5
Hypertension   7
Heart failure   9
Peripheral vascular disease   12
Deep vein thrombosis   13
Ten top tips   15

ANATOMY AT A GLANCE

The basic structure of the heart together with the electrical conducting system is shown in Figure 1.1.

Note that the left atrium drains blood into the left ventricle with the left atrioventricular valve preventing reflux back into the atrium. The right atrioventricular valve prevents blood from regurgitating back into the right atrium from the right ventricle.

PHYSIOLOGY YOU NEED TO KNOW

The *cardiac cycle* is the term used to describe the activity associated with one heart beat and involves the two phases of diastole and systole.

■ Diastole is the resting period during which the two ventricles fill with blood draining under gravity from the atria. During diastole, the right atrium is filled with venous blood from the systemic circulation and the left atrium is filled with oxygenated blood returning from the lungs.

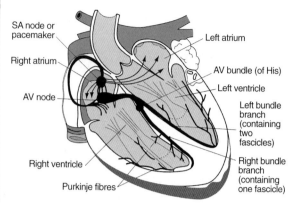

Figure 1.1 The electrical conduction system.

■ Systole corresponds to the powerful contraction of the ventricular muscle which simultaneously sends blood from the right ventricle via the pulmonary arteries to the lungs and from the left ventricle via the aorta around the systemic circulation. The term 'atrial systole' is used to describe contraction of the atria at the end of diastole. This ensures that the ventricles are filled to maximum capacity before systole.

The cardiac cycle is controlled by the conducting mechanism of the heart. Cardiac muscle possesses autorhythmicity, i.e. it initiates its own contractions as a result of a wave of depolarization spreading from the sinoatrial (SA) node through the atria. The rate at which the SA node fires (and hence the heart beats) is governed by many factors of which the activity of the sympathetic and parasympathetic divisions of the autonomic nervous system are the most important, together with the release of the hormones epinephrine and norepinephrine from the medulla of the adrenal glands.

The wave of depolarization initiated by the SA node is picked up by the atrioventricular (AV) node, conducted via the bundle of His, the left and right bundle branches and the spreading network of Purkinje fibres into the ventricular muscle where it initiates ventricular contraction. This electrical activity is recorded as the electrocardiogram (ECG) whose components are as follows:

P wave   SA node discharge and atrial depolarization
PQ interval   Delay while electrical impulse is conducted through conducting fibres
QRS waves   Ventricular contraction
T wave   Repolarization for next heart beat (diastole).

The left and right coronary arteries leave the aorta immediately after the aortic valve and conduct blood to the cardiac muscle. The aorta is the main arterial trunk carrying oxygenated blood via a succession of other arteries to the rest of the body. Venous drainage eventually reaches the heart via the superior and inferior vena cava.

Blood pressure is determined by the strength of the heart beat, volume of blood in the circulation, the elasticity of vessels and the resistance offered to blood passing through blood vessels. Both systolic and diastolic blood pressures are important in assessing hypertension.

ANGINA PECTORIS (P280)

PATHOLOGY: Key facts

Inadequate blood supply to cardiac muscle means there is insufficient oxygen to meet the metabolic needs of muscle during increased activity leading to central chest pain. The cause is usually atheroma, the development of plaques composed of lipids, collagen fibres and smooth muscle cells which narrow the lumen of the coronary artery. Approximately 2 million people in the UK have angina.

WHAT TO LOOK OUT FOR

- Central chest pain upon exertion or during periods of stress which is relieved by rest.
- The pain may radiate to the shoulders, arms, neck or jaw and may not even be felt in the chest at all.
- As the arterial disease process advances, anginal pain becomes more frequent and occurs with less exertion or even at rest; this is unstable angina.

MEDICAL MANAGEMENT

The aim is to balance oxygenated blood supply to the myocardium with demand in order that painful episodes may be avoided. The presence of angina indicates advanced arterial disease which could lead to a more serious and possibly fatal event such as a myocardial infarction (MI) or cerebrovascular accident (CVA). The patient will therefore be investigated and key indicators such as blood pressure and blood lipids monitored regularly. Direct interventions to relieve the symptoms include percutaneous transluminal coronary angioplasty (PTCA) which involves passing a catheter to within the atherosclerotic lesion and then inflating a balloon to stretch the artery, widening the lumen of the artery and increasing blood flow (p282).

PHARMACOLOGY FOCUS

Glyceryl trinitrate (GTN) is the main drug used, this dilates blood vessels reducing the volume of blood returning to the heart (preload) and the diastolic blood pressure against which the heart has to work to pump blood around the body (afterload). As a result the amount of work that the ventricular muscle has to perform is reduced, thereby reducing oxygen demand. It also dilates the coronary arteries, improving blood supply to the myocardium.

PRIORITIES FOR NURSING CARE

- *Health education to focus on*
  - Patient understanding of the cause and meaning of pain.
  - Ensure that patient fully understands use of GTN and coping with acute episodes.
  - Preventive strategies to avoid episodes of angina.
  - Discuss anxieties and fears associated with angina.
- *Lifestyle modification*
  - If needed, weight loss, smoking cessation and alteration to healthier diet.
  - Moderate exercise that will not bring on pain such as walking should be encouraged and built into a supervised programme of increased activity.

- *Primary care*
  - Assess home/family circumstances.
  - Discuss health education and lifestyle modification with carers/family.
  - Ensure that district nurse is involved if necessary.

MYOCARDIAL INFARCTION (P284)

PATHOLOGY: Key facts

Arteriosclerosis of a coronary artery advances to the stage where blood supply to a portion of myocardium is so reduced that the myocardium suffers necrosis through lack of oxygen. This may be associated with the formation of thrombus in advanced complex atherosclerotic lesions which completely occludes the artery at the site of the lesion. Part of the thrombus may break off as an embolism and occlude the arterial lumen further down the artery. The area of necrosed tissue may be small or large and may extend through the full thickness of the ventricular wall. Death can be immediate or within a few hours while survival depends upon the volume of tissue destroyed and its location within the myocardium.

WHAT TO LOOK OUT FOR

- Severe central chest pain, often crushing in nature, unrelieved by GTN.
- Shortness of breath, nausea and possibly vomiting.
- Fatigue and anxiety.
- Pale skin due to reduced cardiac output.
- Low blood pressure.
- There is a potential for cardiac arrhythmias some of which may prove rapidly fatal (ventricular tachycardia or fibrillation).
- Up to 25% of patients may not experience pain and this is known as the 'silent MI'. This is particularly common in older persons.

MEDICAL MANAGEMENT

- Early diagnosis is crucial as most deaths occur within the first hour and prompt treatment to dissolve away the clot in the coronary artery greatly improves the prognosis amongst survivors. A 12-lead ECG should be performed at the earliest opportunity as an elevated ST section is diagnostic of acute MI. Bloods are taken for the presence of certain chemicals known to be in myocardial cells. Their presence in the blood indicates that they have leaked from damaged myocardium and this confirms the diagnosis of MI. Troponin T or I levels rise within a few hours of MI. Myoglobin is another marker for damaged myocardial cells and together with troponin can be measured with a bedside test. The cardiac enzyme creatine phosphokinase (CPK) peaks between 12 and 24 hours while lactic dehydrogenase (LDH) peaks between 3 and 6 days and is useful for a late presentation.

■ Immediate care is concerned with pain relief, myocardial reperfusion and preventing arrhythmias. The patient should therefore be given analgesia and thrombolytic therapy (see below) and placed on continual ECG monitoring. Myocardial workload must immediately be reduced (hence the need for rest) although the patient is mobilized ready for discharge as quickly as possible (see below).

PHARMACOLOGY FOCUS

■ Analgesia (p272): IV diamorphine given slowly at a rate of 1 mg/minute up to 5 minutes followed by a further 2.5–5 mg if needed and an anti-emetic such as prochlorperazine.

■ Thrombolysis therapy (p287) to break down clots, should be given as quickly as possible. Streptokinase and tissue plasminogen activator (tPA) are the most common agents used. Aspirin 300 mg is also given at the same time for its effect in preventing platelet aggregation.

PRIORITIES FOR NURSING CARE (P290)

■ *Acute stage*
  ● Assessment and recognition of cardiac pain followed by prompt initiation of treatment.
  ● Administer oxygen 4–8 L/min.
  ● Rest and quiet stress-free environment.

- Venous cannulation.
- 12-lead ECG and attach to ECG monitor.
- Assist with analgesia and thrombolysis.
- Reassurance and psychological support.
- *Continuing care*
  - Initial bed rest followed by systematic mobilization.
  - ECG/vital signs monitoring.
  - Observe and assess for pain.
  - Maintain quiet environment and offer psychological support to patient and family members.
  - Encourage self care, eating, drinking, etc.
  - Avoid straining (laxatives if needed) and isometric exercise.
- *Rehabilitation*
  - Exercise programme tailored to the needs of the individual.
  - Health education on risk factor modification, lifestyle issues such as smoking, diet, exercise, sexual activity, etc.
  - Psychological support and possibly counselling long term for both patient and partner.

HYPERTENSION (P311)

PATHOLOGY: Key facts

Hypertension means a *sustained* increase in blood pressure (BP). A single elevated reading does not therefore mean a person is hypertensive. There is no simple value above which somebody is said to be hypertensive as the risks increase with increasing BP. If a person's BP is below 140/90 no immediate action is needed unless they have some other disorder such as diabetes or kidney disease; however, treatment guidelines (p312) indicate that as the BP increases above that level the urgency for treatment increases also. Abnormal single readings usually need to be confirmed by subsequent measurements before treatment begins. In approximately 90% of cases no obvious cause for the hypertension can be found and this is called essential or primary hypertension. In the remaining 10% where a cause can be found (often renal) the condition is called secondary hypertension.

WHAT TO LOOK OUT FOR

■ Patients are often unaware that they have raised BP as there are no obvious symptoms although persistent headaches may occur.

■ Over a period of years damage to various organs develops, especially the heart, kidneys and eyes.

■ The hypertensive patient is at much greater risk of a medical emergency such as an MI or CVA.

MEDICAL MANAGEMENT

Antihypertensive drugs (see below) are the mainstay of medical management in moderate to severe cases. Lifestyle modification (weight loss, smoking cessation, dietary improvements such as reducing sodium intake and developing strategies to reduce stress) and careful BP monitoring constitute the principal approach to mild cases.

PHARMACOLOGY FOCUS (P314)

The principal groups of drugs used are:

■ Diuretics such as furosemide or spironolactone.

■ Angiotensin converting enzyme (ACE) inhibitors: these interfere with the conversion of angiotensin I to angiotensin II, a hormone involved in raising blood pressure by causing vasoconstriction and stimulating the release of the hormone aldosterone, which increases the reabsorption of sodium and water in the kidneys.

■ Blocking agents such as the beta blockers which blockade the sympathetic nervous system receptors (e.g. propanolol).

■ Calcium channel blockers (e.g. nifedipine) which reduce the influx of calcium ions into cardiac muscle cells thereby reducing the force of contraction of myocardial cells.

PRIORITIES FOR NURSING CARE

■ *Lifestyle modification*
  ● Many practice nurses (PNs) run their own hypertension clinics in which they advise patients about the key changes they need to make in their lifestyle such as

those outlined above. The PN also teaches the patient about their medication and possible side effects as this may have to be taken for the rest of the person's life and non-adherence to therapy can have serious consequences.

● BP monitoring needs to be carried out regularly at clinic along with regular weighing. Urine may be tested for evidence of developing renal damage, serum creatinine will also be measured to estimate glomerular filtration rate, a key indicator for possible chronic kidney disease.

● Encouragement and psychological support are essential as the patient has to maintain long-term motivation. The family should be fully involved in patient teaching for this reason.

HEART FAILURE (P304)

PATHOLOGY: Key facts

Heart failure is a syndrome in which the heart is unable to provide sufficient cardiac output to keep body tissue adequately perfused. There are various reasons why the heart may gradually fail (chronic heart failure) such as disease of the cardiac muscle, heart valve problems, or abnormally high afterload which means the heart has to work against steadily increasing back pressure. This can be due to severe lung disease (right-sided failure) or hypertension (left-sided failure). Acute heart failure can be caused by an MI which severely weakens cardiac muscle (acute left-sided failure) or a pulmonary embolism (acute right-sided failure). Whichever side of the heart is affected first, failure of both sides usually develops (congestive heart failure) because the function of left and right sides is interdependent. Problems on one side will eventually cause problems on the other. Normally osmotic pressure (which tends to move fluid into the blood vessels) is stronger than the blood pressure within the venous capillaries leading to a net movement of fluid from the interstitial compartment into the capillaries. An increase in venous pressure, associated with a failing heart chamber, unbalances the normal balance of capillary blood and osmotic pressures, inhibiting the movement of fluid back into the venous capillary bed. This leads to fluid accumulation in the affected tissues known as oedema.

WHAT TO LOOK OUT FOR

■ Breathlessness, tiredness and fatigue as the heart cannot meet the body's circulatory requirements.
■ Right-sided failure leads to systemic oedema accumulating (due to gravity) in dependent areas such as the sacrum and lower legs.
■ Acute left-sided failure (typically following an MI) leads to fluid accumulation in the lungs (pulmonary oedema) which makes breathing even more difficult and distressing.
■ Heart failure leads to steady decrease in activity. The person may become housebound, anxious and depressed with significant effects on the rest of the family.

MEDICAL MANAGEMENT

This will focus on two areas, the underlying cause of the heart failure and trying to improve the function of the heart (see below). Often in severe cases, a heart transplant is the only option as the patient's heart is so severely and irretrievably compromised by the disease process (e.g. MI).

PHARMACOLOGY FOCUS

To help the patient, the following main groups of drugs are used:

■ ACE inhibitors such as captopril are the mainstay of treatment. This group of drugs causes vasodilation, thereby reducing systemic and pulmonary vascular resistance. Cardiac output increases but the workload of the heart declines, greatly improving cardiac efficiency.
■ Diuretics reduce fluid retention and are usually combined with ACE inhibitors.
■ Beta-blockers such as bisoprolol and carvedilol may also be used for stable heart failure but only under specialist supervision because of the risk of side effects.

■ Digoxin was the traditional drug used to treat heart failure as it improved cardiac contractility. However, it is only recommended for use today in patients with atrial fibrillation or those who have failed to respond to the above medications.

PRIORITIES FOR NURSING CARE (P307)

■ *Coping with decreased cardiac output*
  ● Ensure that correct medications are given and that patient learns self-medication, including knowledge of side effects.
  ● Administer oxygen if needed.
  ● Promotion of rest and physical comfort. Take measures to avoid risks of immobilization such as deep vein thrombosis (DVT), chest infection, pressure sores.
  ● Position sitting upright to facilitate breathing.
  ● Avoid constipation. This is distressing and straining puts extra workload on the heart.
■ *Fluid volume excess*
  ● Correct administration of diuretic coupled with accurate fluid balance.
  ● Regular weighing.
  ● May require fluid and/or dietary sodium restriction.
  ● Provide convenience and privacy for micturition.
■ *Anxiety*
  ● Help patient accept reality of the situation and allow the person to talk about their feelings.
  ● Be honest and realistic.
  ● Include family in discussion.
■ *Lifestyle modification*
  ● This may include smoking cessation, weight reduction, dietary modification and developing an activity plan. However, check patient is well enough to understand what is being said and is able to engage in any health education before attempting such.
  ● Include family in discussions.
  ● Plan discharge and continuing support and care in community which may include domestic rearrangements such as sleeping downstairs, selling the family home or going into a care home. The potential of such

major changes may be very distressing and lead to much anxiety.

PERIPHERAL VASCULAR DISEASE (P316)

PATHOLOGY: Key facts

Atherosclerosis and arteriosclerosis of the arteries supplying the lower limbs leads to a progressive decrease in blood supply. Eventually, small areas of necrotic tissue appear on the foot or heel which may then become infected. They may be associated with a minor injury or may occur spontaneously. Amputation of the lower limb is usually required in advanced cases such as this. The disease is associated with all the risk factors for vascular disease particularly diabetes.

WHAT TO LOOK OUT FOR

- Intermittent claudication or pain on exercise in the calf muscle. As the blood supply diminishes, insufficient oxygen reaches the calf muscle leading to the metabolic build up of lactic acid which causes the pain and spasm of intermittent claudication.
- Rest relieves the pain. However, as the disease progresses, the person notices they can walk shorter and shorter distances before the pain comes on.
- Continual and severe pain in advanced cases.
- The affected limb is colder and the skin discoloured whilst peripheral pulses become weak and disappear.

MEDICAL MANAGEMENT

Careful investigation is necessary to locate the blockage and to show the degree of circulatory impairment. This involves techniques such as Doppler ultrasound, angiography and measuring the ratio of ankle to brachial systolic blood pressures (Ankle Brachial Pressure Index). Treatment usually involves surgery to bypass the narrowed artery with a Teflon or Dacron graft. In the meantime, lifestyle modification such as giving up smoking and the control of other disease processes such as diabetes are essential. Amputation of the limb may ultimately be necessary (p850).

PHARMACOLOGY FOCUS

Drug therapy has made little impact upon the problem of peripheral vascular disease.

PRIORITIES FOR NURSING CARE

- Lifestyle modification involves smoking cessation, weight loss and adapting to reduced activity tolerance.
- The patient should be encouraged to manage other health problems such as diabetes which often coexist with peripheral vascular disease (PVD).
- Motivation, family involvement and psychological support are essential as the patient will have to face major surgery with the possibility of ultimately losing a limb. Depression and refusal to face reality will lead to a much worse outcome than a willingness to try and make the best of things.
- Preparation for surgery .
- Management of patient after amputation (p852).

DEEP VEIN THROMBOSIS (P319)

PATHOLOGY: Key facts

A DVT is a blood clot affecting one of the deep veins of the leg, usually caused by venous stasis. The main danger is that if a piece of the clot breaks free it will be carried to the right side of the heart via the inferior vena cava and will be pumped directly to the lungs. Here it will occlude one of the pulmonary arteries (pulmonary embolism, or PE), which is potentially fatal if the embolism is big enough and lodges in a major artery. In this scenario, a large section of lung has effectively been deprived of its blood supply.

WHAT TO LOOK OUT FOR

- Localized tenderness and pain in the calf (especially on walking).
- The affected calf may feel warmer and there may be evidence of swelling.

■ A major PE is a medical emergency causing sudden chest pain, severe shortness of breath and collapse requiring urgent attempts at resuscitation.

■ A smaller embolism will lead to breathlessness, pain, haemoptysis and an elevated temperature.

MEDICAL MANAGEMENT

DVT is difficult to diagnose on physical examination alone so careful medical investigations are required involving D-dimer testing, contrast venography and compression ultrasonography. Anticoagulation therapy is instituted rapidly (see below).

If the patient suffers a major PE, full-scale resuscitation may be necessary. The diagnosis of PE may only be made at post-mortem.

PHARMACOLOGY FOCUS

A bolus dose of heparin (5000 units) is given once the diagnosis of DVT has been made, followed by either a heparin infusion or subcutaneous low molecular weight heparin. Heparin prevents clot enlargement whilst natural solution of the clot takes place. Warfarin is an oral anticoagulant (heparin cannot be given orally) but it takes 3 days to become fully effective. It is started immediately the patient is diagnosed. Dosage is adjusted according to the international normalized ratio (INR), which is a measure of clotting established from the prothrombin time. An INR in the range 2–3 is the target.

PRIORITIES FOR NURSING CARE

Prevention of DVT is the main priority. Once a DVT has occurred, elevation, graded compression stockings and early mobilization are very helpful. Practice nurses and nurse practitioners regularly manage many DVT patients in the community, monitoring their INR and adjusting medication accordingly together with the GP.

TEN TOP TIPS

1. Always ensure that chest pain is promptly reported to a senior nurse, lie the patient down, give oxygen and psychological support.
2. Make sure you know the ward/health centre resuscitation drill and location of all resuscitation equipment.
3. Follow correct procedures at all times for measuring BP, do not take short cuts.
4. Remember that cardiovascular problems cause a great deal of anxiety amongst patients and family; offer psychological support.
5. Health education about lifestyle modification can pay enormous dividends if it turns into alterations in behaviour such as weight reduction, smoking cessation, dietary changes and increased levels of exercise.
6. Cardiovascular disorders are long-term health problems that require continual management after discharge from hospital. Carry out a reality check in light of home circumstances on what you are teaching the patient.
7. Ensure good communication with GP, PN and primary care team.
8. Cardiovascular drugs are very potent and have potentially serious unwanted effects, therefore ensure that the patient is fully aware of the side-effects of their medication and understands their drug regime.
9. Remember convenience and privacy for passing urine if patient is on diuretics.
10. If the patient is on a daily weighing regime, ensure that the scales are regularly checked, and that the patient wears similar clothes at each weighing.

2

Caring for the patient with respiratory problems

Anatomy at a glance   17
Physiology you need to know   17
Chronic obstructive pulmonary disease (COPD)   20
Asthma   23
Pneumonia   25
Pulmonary tuberculosis   29
Respiratory failure   31
Ten top tips   33

ANATOMY AT A GLANCE

The basic structure of the respiratory system is summarized for you in Figure 2.1. Refer to this diagram whilst reading about the physiology in the next section.

PHYSIOLOGY YOU NEED TO KNOW

■ *Pulmonary ventilation* is the movement of air into and out of the lungs. It is carried out by increasing the volume of the thorax on inspiration thereby reducing pressure within the lungs to less than atmospheric. At rest this is accomplished by the diaphragm being lowered 1 cm which is sufficient to pull in some 500 mL of air. Exercise requires greater volumes of air to be inhaled. Contraction of the external intercostal and shoulder muscles further increases the volume of the thorax as the chest wall moves upwards and outwards, reducing pressure further and drawing larger volumes of air into the lungs. Expiration is a passive process of elastic recoil aided by the action of

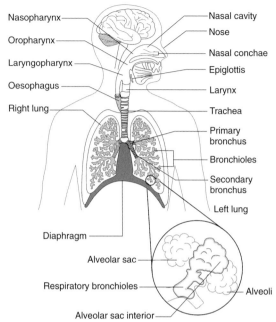

Figure 2.1 The respiratory system.

the internal intercostal muscles pulling the chest wall inwards during exertion.

Normal ventilation depends upon airways called bronchioles which have the capacity to adjust their cross-sectional area due to the presence of smooth muscle tissue in their walls. Bronchioles branch off from the main bronchi and conduct air to the small alveoli where gas exchange occurs.

■ *External respiration* is the gas exchange taking place within the alveoli. Oxygen diffuses across the very thin respiratory membrane of each alveolus from atmospheric air into the pulmonary capillaries. Carbon dioxide moves in the opposite direction. Both gases move down their partial pressure gradients.

- *Internal respiration.* This term describes the movement of gases between the capillaries of the systemic circulation and tissue cells. This occurs by diffusion down partial pressure gradients with O_2 entering cells and CO_2 entering the capillaries.

- *Cellular respiration* occurs within cells and involves the manufacture of adenosine triphosphate (ATP) within the mitochondria of the cell. ATP is the source of energy which drives cellular metabolism. Its manufacture requires glucose to enter the cell and be converted to pyruvic acid which is then fed into the Krebs Cycle, a complex piece of organic chemistry, to produce ATP. This can only operate in the presence of oxygen and produces water and carbon dioxide as waste products, which the cell has to dispose of.

- *Oxygen transport* within the blood depends upon haemoglobin (Hb) which readily combines with oxygen molecules to form a molecule of oxyhaemoglobin. This molecule readily dissociates and releases oxygen molecules. When Hb has combined with all the oxygen it can it is said to be saturated. The degree of saturation of Hb is measured by a pulse oximeter and depends largely upon the amount of oxygen present in the blood as measured by its partial pressure. Oxygen saturation readings are therefore a good guide to the amount of oxygen available in the bloodstream and the aim should always be to keep them over 95%.

- *Carbon dioxide transport* is more complex. Some CO_2 is dissolved in plasma (7%) and some is attached to haemoglobin as carbaminohaemoglobin (23%). The remaining 70% is carried as bicarbonate ions (HCO_3^-) which combine with hydrogen ions in the lungs to form CO_2 (exhaled) and H_2O.

- *Blood pH* reflects the degree of acidity of the blood as measured by the concentration of hydrogen ions. Arterial blood pH is normally in the range 7.35–7.45. A figure below that is called acidosis and if this is caused by respiratory problems such as CO_2 retention, this is called respiratory acidosis. Metabolic acidosis indicates the cause is metabolic such as a diabetic ketoacidotic state.

CHRONIC OBSTRUCTIVE PULMONARY DISEASE (COPD) (P337)

PATHOLOGY: Key facts

- *COPD* is a term that covers several different diseases such as chronic bronchitis, emphysema and bronchiectasis. Patients are usually elderly and have a history of smoking for many years which has greatly contributed to the disease process. As the term COPD implies, the person is suffering from a slowly progressive airway obstruction which leads to a gradual deterioration in ventilation and gas exchange such that the person can no longer meet their body requirements for oxygen. Gradually respiratory failure develops.

- *Chronic bronchitis* is caused by hyperactivity of the mucus secreting glands that line the bronchial mucosa. Overgrowth of the glands (hyperplasia) coupled with the increased volumes of secretions narrow the airway passages. Infection of retained secretions commonly leads to recurring chest infections. The original cause of the problem is mainly the irritants in cigarette smoke and possibly atmospheric pollution.

- *Emphysema* involves the destruction of alveolar walls and elastic tissue. There is therefore a loss of lung volume available for gas exchange and compliance within the lung (the lung becomes 'stiffer'). Cigarette smoke is the main cause. Emphysema and chronic bronchitis frequently occur in the same person and may be complicated by the presence of asthma (see below).

- *Bronchiectasis* is a term used to describe abnormal dilation of the bronchi. In adults it is frequently caused by the accumulation of pus beyond a lesion which is obstructing a bronchus such as a bronchial carcinoma. It is seen in people with cystic fibrosis as a result of the accumulation of thick mucus and recurrent infections and may also be secondary to serious lung diseases such as suppurative pneumonia or pulmonary tuberculosis. Chronic inflammatory changes occur together with the accumulation of pus within the cavities that form leading to coughing, copious production of purulent sputum and a general deterioration in the patient's condition.

WHAT TO LOOK OUT FOR

- Respiratory failure, therefore respiratory rate and depth should be carefully monitored along with other vital signs.
- Monitor oxygen saturation levels using pulse oximetry.
- Level of consciousness as deteriorating respiratory function will lead eventually to cerebral hypoxia, confusion and disorientation.
- Signs of agitation and anxiety leading to lethargy and drowsiness also suggest cerebral hypoxia.
- Sputum for signs of blood or pus.
- Cyanosis is a late sign of respiratory failure.
- Exercise tolerance and breathlessness should be monitored. Exercise tolerance gradually decreases with advancing disease to the point where even just walking across the room leaves the person breathless and distressed.
- Psychological factors should also be considered as the person may be very frightened during acute breathlessness and feel depressed at their incapacity and continual struggle for breath.

MEDICAL MANAGEMENT

Smoking cessation is essential. Respiratory infections will be treated vigorously with antimicrobial drugs as they exacerbate breathlessness. Short-acting β_2 agonists such as salbutamol delivered by inhalers are helpful because of their bronchodilator effect. Exercise is important while improvements in diet and if obese, weight loss, will assist greatly. Patients with severe disease benefit from long-term oxygen therapy at home, 2 L/minute delivered by nasal cannulae.

PHARMACOLOGY FOCUS

Short-acting β_2 agonists such as salbutamol and terbutaline are helpful for symptom relief. If symptoms are persistent in more serious cases then an antimuscarinic bronchodilator such as ipratropium will be used. This group of drugs are considered more effective in treating COPD than asthma. Antimicrobial therapy is discussed elsewhere, but generally amoxicillin is prescribed for exacerbations of chronic bronchitis.

PRIORITIES FOR NURSING CARE

The overall aim is to help the patient achieve effective respiration so that greater levels of activity can be maintained.

- *Respiratory support* involves helping the patient with an acute episode of breathlessness by positioning (sitting upright to maximize chest expansion) and coaching the patient in slower deeper respirations whilst providing psychological support. Close cooperation with the physiotherapist is essential to help with breathing exercises and pulmonary rehabilitation. Always check that oxygen cannulae are in place and are delivering the required flow rate.
- *Activity* needs to be carefully planned to avoid exhausting the patient. Both the physiotherapist and occupational therapist have important roles to play in rehabilitation and discharge planning. Coping strategies and personal preferences that have developed over the years need to be respected by the nurse. Inactivity increases the risk of pressure sores, DVT and further chest infections. It is also demoralizing for the person.
- *Hydration and nutrition* need to be carefully supervised and encouraged. The patient may be mouth breathing which will lead to a dry and unpleasant mouth. Dehydration will lead to thicker body secretions including mucus within the lung, consequently it is necessary to encourage fluid intake. A healthy diet should be planned with the dietician and provided for the patient. If obese, weight loss will assist the patient in coping although with severely limited activity this will be difficult to achieve.
- *Patient and family teaching* leading to maximum self care after discharge is essential. This will cover the need to stop smoking and if appropriate, weight loss. Coping strategies to balance the activity the patient is capable of, with their needs, should be developed. Education about medication,

its correct administration using an inhaler and long-term oxygen therapy is needed.

■ *Psychological support*, stimulation and motivation will help greatly as the person may become depressed and socially isolated by their inactivity.

■ *Liaison* with the primary health care team should take place well before discharge. The vast majority of care for patients with COPD is provided by the Primary Health Care Team (PHCT) and informal carers.

ASTHMA (P338)

PATHOLOGY: Key facts

Asthma is a syndrome involving inflammation of the bronchi, hyperresponsiveness of the airway and airway obstruction that is usually reversible. Childhood asthma is common and often related to allergens but frequently abates as the child grows. Adult onset asthma is often not recognized as such for some time and tends to be more permanent. Because the airways are overresponsive, an agent that would not cause a health problem in other people can provoke an asthmatic attack in a susceptible person. The agent produces oedema and thickening of the mucosa, hypersecretion of the mucus glands within the airways and spasmodic contractions of the smooth muscle in the wall of the airways. The net effect is narrowing of the airway and plugging with mucus which makes expiration very difficult leading to the classic wheeze and shortness of breath associated with asthma.

WHAT TO LOOK OUT FOR

■ Difficulty in breathing.
■ Tight feeling in the chest.
■ Wheeze.
■ Anxiety (asthma is a frightening experience).
■ In moderate to severe episodes the person sits upright and uses their accessory muscles of respiration.
■ In severe cases the pulse can be 110, respiratory rate 25 and peak expiratory flow rate (PEFR) 50% of normal.

■ It is impossible to complete sentences because of shortness of breath.

■ In serious life-threatening episodes the patient may appear very still, look exhausted, be unable to speak and make little respiratory effort. There will be no obvious wheeze. This indicates that their respiratory obstruction is nearly complete and constitutes a life-threatening emergency. Blood pressure will be low and pulse rate rapid, PEFR will be less than 33% of normal and cyanosis may be apparent. Respiratory arrest is imminent.

■ At the other extreme however, the presentation may be little more than a persistent cough that is keeping the patient awake at night, leading to the person attending their GP.

MEDICAL MANAGEMENT

This is usually carried out in the community but an acute exacerbation may lead to urgent hospital admission. For a severe episode initial treatment involves oxygen 40–60%, salbutamol 5 mg via an oxygen driven nebulizer and either prednisolone (30–60 mg orally) or hydrocortisone (200 mg IV). The patient must be closely monitored at all times with PEFR taken before and after treatment and continual pulse oximetry.

Management in primary care follows the British Thoracic Society Guidelines with the emphasis on prevention via the use of inhaled corticosteroids. This reduces the need for the symptomatic relief provided by short-acting beta$_2$-agonist drugs such as salbutamol.

PHARMACOLOGY FOCUS

Corticosteroids have an anti-inflammatory effect and therefore should be used regularly to prevent episodes. The beta$_2$-agonists cause rapid bronchodilation by stimulating sympathetic nervous system receptor sites in the bronchioles. A further group of drugs that have been introduced into treatment are the leucotriene receptor agonists (montelukasts) which have an anti-inflammatory effect. They are useful for helping patients with mild to moderate asthma where corticosteroids and b$_2$-agonists are insufficient to control symptoms.

PRIORITIES FOR NURSING CARE

During an acute episode you should seek assistance from senior staff immediately. The patient should then be:

- Sat upright if possible.
- Given high-concentration oxygen (40–60%).
- Reassured and encouraged to try and breath more deeply and steadily.
- Assessed carefully for danger signs (see Figure 2.2).
- Treated in accordance with flow charts (Figures 2.2 and 2.3).
- Not left alone until situation is resolved.

Health education is very important, especially teaching the patient and family to recognize the early warnings of an asthmatic attack. They should be taught to monitor PEFR at regular intervals and to be aware of any trend such as a gradual reduction in PEFR which may herald an acute episode. The person should also be taught the correct use of medication. Corticosteroids to prevent attacks ('preventers') should be encouraged, particularly as repeated use of drugs used to produce rapid relief from symptoms ('relievers') such as salbutamol may be harmful. Drugs that are contra-indicated for people with asthma such as the non-steroidal anti-inflammatory drugs (NSAIDs) should also be discussed together with factors that bring on attacks so that avoidance strategies can be worked out. Smoking is to be particularly discouraged.

PNEUMONIA (P334)

PATHOLOGY: Key facts

Pneumonia involves infection and inflammation of the lung tissue which produces shadowing on the chest radiograph. The alveoli become filled with fluid and blood cells making gas exchange very difficult, leading to shortness of breath.

Immediate treatment

Oxygen 40–60%
Salbutamol 5 mg or terbutaline
10 mg by oxygen-driven nebulizer
Prednisolone 30–60 mg orally
or hydrocortisone 200 mg
intravenously
No sedation
Chest radiograph

Life-threatening features

- Peak flow <33% predicted or best
- Silent chest, feeble respiratory effort
- Cyanosis
- Bradycardia, hypotension
- Exhaustion, confusion, coma
- $P_{CO_2} \geq 5$ kPa, $P_{O_2} \leq 8$ kPa, acidosis

If life-threatening features are present

Add ipratropium bromide 0.5 mg to nebulizer
Aminophylline 250 mg intravenously or
salbutamol or terbutaline 250 µg intravenously

Improving

Continue
oxygen
Prednisolone 30–60 mg daily
β-agonist at least 4 hourly

Not improving after 15–30 minutes

Continue
oxygen and steroids
β-agonist up to every 15 minutes
Ipratropium bromide
0.5 mg 2–6 hourly

If still not improving

Aminophylline infusion 0.5 mg/kg·hour
(monitor concentrations if longer than 24 hours)
or
salbutamol or terbutaline infusion 5–15 µg/min

Monitor

- Peak flow before and after nebulizations
- Oximetry (keep saturation >92%)
- Blood gas tensions if initial PaO_2 <8 kPa and saturation <93% or $PaCO_2$ normal or high or patient deteriorates

Figure 2.2 Treatment of acute severe asthma in hospital.

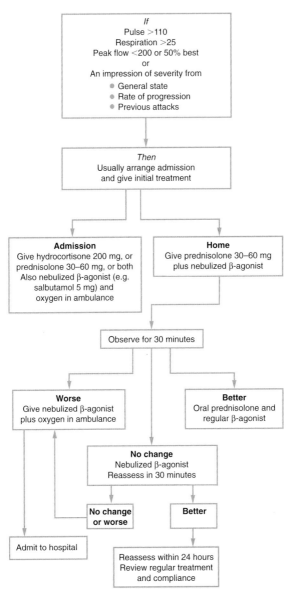

Figure 2.3 Treatment of acute severe asthma in primary care.

Pneumonia is classified as either hospital or community acquired. Pneumococci are a common cause of the condition but a range of bacteria and viruses may also cause pneumonia. A hospital-acquired infection is much more difficult to treat because of the increased risk of antibiotic resistance. Immunocompromised patients (e.g. acquired immune deficiency syndrome, or AIDS) are another important group of patients who may develop pneumonia. Owing to the development of antibiotic resistance, pneumonia is classified into community or hospital acquired categories. The latter is usually much more difficult to treat for this reason.

WHAT TO LOOK OUT FOR

Onset may be very sudden and the outcome may be fatal.

- Elderly patients who are already immobilized and debilitated as a result of other serious health problems tend to have a slower onset but a higher mortality rate as they are prone to developing hypostatic pneumonia. This term refers to lack of mobility/accumulation of secretions in the lung leading to increased risk of infection.
- Increasing pulse rate and respiratory rate together with a fever are common signs of a developing pneumonia.
- The patient feels tired and unwell.
- Breathing becomes painful leading to shallow respirations and a cough develops.
- Sputum is produced which may be blood stained, rust coloured and/or purulent.
- In older persons the presentation may initially be increased confusion (caused by cerebral hypoxia) associated with incontinence and lethargy.

MEDICAL MANAGEMENT

A chest radiograph and a sputum sample for culture and sensitivity are urgently required to confirm the diagnosis and identify the causative organism. Bloods will also be taken for culture and serology. Antimicrobial therapy should be commenced as soon as possible with general supportive measures to ensure adequate hydration, nutrition and elimination.

PHARMACOLOGY FOCUS

Antimicrobial therapy can bring about a dramatic improvement in the patient's condition if the causative organism is sensitive to the drug used. However if it is resistant, the patient will not improve. The patient's condition may be so serious that delay waiting for the results of sensitivity tests is not possible. Inappropriate antimicrobial therapy only increases the risk of more bacterial resistance developing. Modern antibiotics are increasingly expensive, however, the most expensive antibiotic of all is the one that does not work. As a result of these factors, most hospitals have developed their own protocols for treating pneumonia. Typically an uncomplicated community-acquired pneumonia is treated with amoxicillin or benzylpenicillin and if *Staphylococcus* is suspected, flucloxacillin is added. Hospital-acquired pneumonia is treated with a broad spectrum antibiotic such as a cephalosporin (e.g. cefotaxime) or an antipseudomonal penicillin such as piperacillin.

PRIORITIES FOR NURSING CARE

Patients will require intensive nursing care during the acute phase of the illness. Oxygen therapy (60%) and upright positioning to assist ventilation are essential together with frequent vital signs monitoring. Hydration and nutrition require particular attention together with reinforcing the work of the physiotherapist to try and clear secretions from the chest if the patient is able to cooperate with treatment. Level of consciousness should be monitored as cerebral hypoxia can cause confusion and disorientation. Pressure areas should be checked regularly, especially in older patients.

PULMONARY TUBERCULOSIS (P344)

PATHOLOGY: Key facts

The tubercle bacillus is responsible for tuberculosis (TB) and while it may attack a wide range of organs in the body, the lungs are the most common sites of infection in Europe. TB has long been recognized as a disease of poverty being most active where people have poor health and living conditions. Worldwide the World Health Organization (WHO) reported over 1.5 million deaths from TB in 2005 with Africa and Southeast Asia being worst affected. In the UK most cases occur amongst people from those ethnic backgrounds. Children and adolescents are at greatest risk. Initial infection is confined to tubercles within the lung, areas full of leucocytes and phagocytes which are fighting the invading organisms. The infection may be successfully eradicated by the body's defence system or may lie dormant within the tubercle and the person will show a positive tubeculin test several weeks later. If the body's defence system is weakened, the dormant organisms can become active and full-scale active TB develops. The tubercle ruptures discharging soft caseous material and leaving a cavity within the lung. This material is highly infective.

WHAT TO LOOK OUT FOR

- While the disease is localized within the lungs it produces a cough, sputum, haemoptysis, shortness of breath.
- If the pleura becomes involved this leads to chest pain.
- Systemic effects include lethargy, malaise, weight loss, appetite loss, low-grade fever towards evening, tachycardia and night sweats.

MEDICAL MANAGEMENT

Diagnosis depends upon tuberculin testing, sputum culture and a chest radiograph. Definitive treatment is by chemotherapy (see below).

PHARMACOLOGY FOCUS

Patients can continue to live at home whilst taking a combination of antimicrobial drugs over a prolonged period of time. Treatment usually starts with an initial 2-month course of pyrazinamide, isoniazid and rifampicin to kill as many bacteria as possible followed by isoniazid and rifampicin only for a further 4 months. Longer periods of treatment as well as the use of other drugs will be needed if the organisms are resistant to the standard antibiotics.

It is essential that the patient completes the full drug regime which may require a great deal of work by the primary care team given the length of time involved and the sometimes difficult home circumstances of some patients. These drugs have potentially harmful side effects such as hypersensitivity reactions whilst rifampicin can interact with other drugs (e.g. oral contraceptives, warfarin) because it is a potent liver enzyme inducer. Continual monitoring for side effects is essential.

PRIORITIES FOR NURSING CARE

In hospital settings infection control procedures should be adhered to at all times and the occupational health department consulted if there is any doubt. Patients are usually managed in the community and cultural awareness is crucial to achieve cooperation in the lengthy course of medication needed. The emergence of antibiotic-resistant strains of the tubercle bacillus owing to ineffective compliance with treatment regimes is a major concern.

RESPIRATORY FAILURE (P352)

PATHOLOGY: Key facts

This term denotes a situation where the patient is unable to maintain normal arterial blood gas levels of oxygen and carbon dioxide. It is defined as an arterial partial oxygen pressure $(PaO_2) < 8.0$ kPa or 60 mmHg or an arterial partial carbon dioxide pressure $(PaCO_2) > 6.2$ kPa or 45 mmHg. This can be caused by many disorders other than respiratory problems such as asthma or COPD. Trauma, shock, sepsis, central nervous system disorder and neuromuscular disease are the common causes. Whatever the disease process, the end product is usually either inadequate ventilation of the alveoli, inadequate gas exchange across the respiratory membrane within the alveoli or lack of blood reaching the lungs to be oxygenated.

WHAT TO LOOK OUT FOR

- Rapid respiratory rate and shortness of breath.
- Alternatively slow, shallow respirations occur if there is central nervous system depression.
- Pulse rate is typically rapid.
- Cerebral hypoxia leads to disorientation and confusion.
- The condition may develop rapidly over a few hours or insidiously over days and weeks.

MEDICAL MANAGEMENT

Immediate treatment is concerned with improving oxygenation of the blood by improving ventilation and oxygen therapy. Bronchodilator drugs, suctioning of the airway, physiotherapy and prompt treatment of any chest infection all help improve ventilation. The underlying cause of the problem must be identified and appropriate treatment instituted as quickly as possible. Close monitoring of blood chemistry and oxygen saturations together with vital signs are essential as the patient may deteriorate to the point where artificial ventilation has to be considered.

PHARMACOLOGY FOCUS

There is much debate about the concentration of oxygen that should be administered to patients with chronic respiratory disease. This stems from the fact that the person has probably become accustomed to a high $PaCO_2$ level and is therefore relying upon low oxygen levels to stimulate breathing. Administering 60% oxygen could therefore theoretically induce respiratory arrest by removing that stimulus. The exact concentration of oxygen that is required should therefore be carefully checked with medical staff.

PRIORITIES FOR NURSING CARE

Close observation, pulse oximetry and monitoring of vital signs including respiratory rate and depth should be combined with careful checking of the flow rate and concentration required for oxygen therapy. Always ensure that tubing is connected and that the mask or nasal cannulae are in place. Note that confusion and disorientation are common due to cerebral hypoxia. Other priorities will depend upon the cause of the patient's respiratory failure.

TEN TOP TIPS

1. Assist patient to sit in an upright position to facilitate chest expansion and breathing.
2. Ensure that you know where the oxygen cylinders/wall points are and that they are stocked with tubing and masks.
3. When a patient is on oxygen therapy, check that the tubing is connected to the source and that the delivery system is correctly placed on the patient's face.
4. Being short of breath is a frightening experience so offer psychological support at all times.
5. Always record respiratory rate and depth, even if only as a baseline measurement on admission.
6. If a patient is short of breath, keep questions short and preferably closed so that they can be answered with a nod of the head.
7. Learn correct inhaler technique so that you can teach patients.
8. Follow closely what the physiotherapist is teaching the patient so that you can reinforce that teaching and ensure that exercises are correct even when the physiotherapist is not present.
9. Remember that the majority of patients with respiratory disease are managed at home by the PHCT so ensure that there is good discharge planning and liaison.
10. Lose no opportunity to encourage smoking cessation and if you smoke yourself, consider what kind of a role model you are (do as I say not as I do?).

Caring for the patient with a haematological disorder

Anatomy at a glance   35
Physiology you need to know   38
Anaemia   40
Leukaemia   44
Malignant lymphomas   47
Ten top tips   49

ANATOMY AT A GLANCE

The haematological system consists of the blood and the sites of blood production (especially red bone marrow and lymphatic tissue). The main components of blood are shown in Figure 3.1. Different types of blood cell all develop from their common origin, the pluripotent stem cell. Red blood cells (RBCs), for example, follow a pathway from the pluripotent stem cell via the myeloid stem cell stage, develop into a proerythroblast, then a reticulocyte when they expel their nucleus to finally become a mature RBC or erythrocyte. The pathways followed by other types of blood cell are shown in Figure 3.2.

SOME KEY NORMAL VALUES FOR BLOOD

Blood volume:	Male 75 mL/kg (average 75 kg male has approx 5 L blood)
	Female 70 mL/kg (average 55–60 kg female has approx 4 L blood)
Haemoglobin:	Male 130–180 g/L
	Female 115–165 g/L

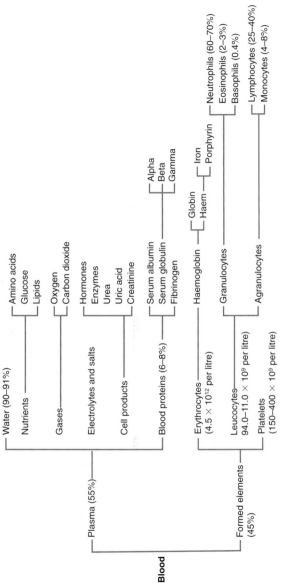

Figure 3.1 Composition of blood.

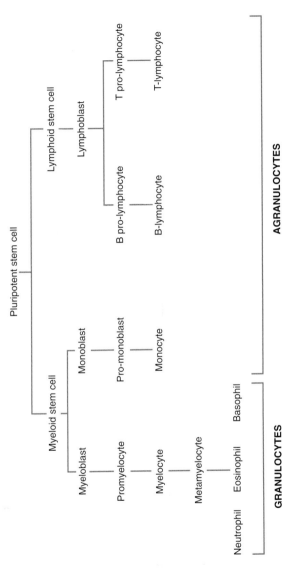

Figure 3.2 Formation of white blood cells (leucopoiesis).

Red cell count:	Male 4.5–6.5 3 1012/L
	Female 3.8–5.8 3 1012/L
Mean lifespan of RBC	120 days
Platelets	150–400 g/L
Leucocytes	4.0–11.0 3 109 g/L
Erythrocyte	Male 0–5 mm/hour
Sedimentation Rate:	Female 0–7 mm/hour
Prothrombin Time	12–14 seconds.

PHYSIOLOGY YOU NEED TO KNOW

MAIN FUNCTIONS OF BLOOD

■ Transport medium for metabolic requirements (e.g. oxygen, nutrients, hormones) and waste products of metabolism (e.g. carbon dioxide).

■ Maintains homeostasis by facilitating regulation of body function, e.g. continual exchange of constituents across capillary wall between blood and interstitial fluid, regulates body temperature by distributing heat around the body.

■ Protection: ingest and destroy (phagocytosis) foreign particles, antibody production mediated by different types of white blood cells, clotting mechanism to prevent bleeding.

CONSTITUENTS OF BLOOD

■ Erythrocytes (RBCs) are biconcave, circular discs with no nucleus. They are packed with haemoglobin whose main function is to carry oxygen and some carbon dioxide. A haemoglobin molecule consists of a protein called globin and a pigment called haem, which contains iron. The more oxygen is attached to the molecule, the redder the colour appears. Four oxygen molecules combine with each haemoglobin molecule to form oxyhaemoglobin which can readily disassociate back into oxygen and haemoglobin when required.

■ Leucocytes (white blood cells). There are three main types:

1. *Granulocytes*

   Neutrophils; phagocytose microbes

   Eosinophils; phagocytose antigen/antibody complexes and attack parasitic worms.

   Basophils intensify inflammatory response by developing into mast cells and releasing histamine, serotonin and heparin.

2. *Lymphocytes*

   B Lymphocytes secrete antibodies to attack antigens. Some B cells serve as memory B cells for future defensive actions against the same antigen.

   T Lymphocytes exist in various forms and attack antigens. Memory T cells can recognize the same antigen and subsequently trigger a powerful defensive response.

3. *Monocytes* differentiate into macrophages which can phagocytose invading organisms.

■ Platelets contain a range of active chemicals and play an important role in stopping haemorrhage by adhering to the injured area. They are derived from the fragmentation of cells called megakaryocytes. They also adhere together to form platelet plugs which help occlude damaged blood vessels and prevent blood loss. This mechanism takes place alongside the clotting mechanism in blood which converts the soluble plasma protein fibrinogen into strands of insoluble fibrin, forming a clot which, together with the platelet plug and localized vasoconstriction, all combine to stop bleeding from severed blood vessels.

■ Plasma is the straw-coloured liquid component of blood which is mostly water but which also contains a range of important solutes (sodium, potassium, etc.) and plasma proteins such as albumin, fibrinogen and gamma globulin antibodies.

■ Blood Groups. Erythrocytes contain on their surface complex molecules known as isoantigens or agglutinogens which act as antigens. These isoantigens occur in characteristic combinations which give rise to a complex series of different blood groups. The original discovery of this system led to the following simple model based upon four possibilities:

Type A antigens	Group A
Type B antigens	Group B
No antigens	Group O
A and B antigens	Group AB

Plasma also contains antibodies or agglutinens which will react with certain antigens:

Anti-A-antibody (plasma) reacts with Antigen A (erythrocyte).

Anti-B-antibody (plasma) reacts with Antigen B (erythrocyte).

A person does not possess the antibody that will react with the antigen they display on their own erythrocytes. Grouping and cross matching for blood transfusion ensures that a person only receives blood that is compatible with their own antibodies so that a potentially fatal antigen–antibody reaction does not occur. Blood group O is known as the universal donor because it does not display any antigens which can provoke an antigen–antibody reaction. Research has shown that there are many different types of blood beyond the basic four types originally described in the ABO system, making grouping and cross matching an essential but time-consuming laboratory procedure.

ANAEMIA (P374)

PATHOLOGY: Key facts

The term anaemia indicates a reduction in the oxygen carrying capacity of the blood and it occurs because of a reduction in the numbers of erythrocytes or a decrease in the concentration of haemoglobin. This results from the body not producing enough erythrocytes or losing/destroying erythrocytes faster than they can be replaced.

1. Inadequate erythrocyte production (erythropoiesis) (p375)
   - Iron deficiency anaemia produces smaller than normal erythrocytes with reduced quantities of haemoglobin. It can not only be caused by a poor diet, but also by chronic blood loss (menstruation, peptic ulcers),

inadequate absorption of iron in the bowel or extra demand for iron exceeding dietary intake as in pregnancy.

- Pernicious anaemia is caused by a lack of absorption of vitamin B_{12} or a deficiency in the diet (notably in vegans) leading to fewer erythrocytes than normal being formed which are, however, bigger than normal (megaloblastic anaemia).
- Folic acid deficiency anaemia is associated with poor diet (alcoholism, anorexia) or malabsorption (Crohn's disease, coeliac disease).
- Vitamin C deficiency caused by poor diet will not only produce scurvy but also anaemia.
- Other abnormalities associated with decreased erythrocyte production include leukaemia and aplastic anaemia.
- Abnormal erythrocyte destruction (haemolytic anaemia) (p378).
- Inherited haemolytic anaemia. A range of genetic disorders can lead to abnormally high rates of destruction of red blood cells such as thalassaemia and sickle cell disease.
- Acquired haemolytic anaemia can be either caused by an immune system problem or in response to various drugs (e.g. salazopyrin), chemicals (e.g. copper, lead poisoning) or severe infections (e.g. malaria).

WHAT TO LOOK OUT FOR

The symptoms and signs of anaemia are outlined in Figure 3.3.

MEDICAL MANAGEMENT

The treatment of anaemia is directed towards discovering and treating where possible the actual cause. This is particularly important where chronic bleeding is suspected, leading to iron deficiency anaemia. Iron supplements will also be required. Vitamin B_{12} or folic acid deficiency anaemias can be treated with replacement therapy as outlined below. Management of haemolytic anaemia depends upon managing the underlying disorder, such as sickle cell disease

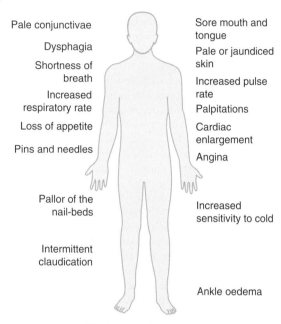

Figure 3.3 Symptoms and signs of anaemia.

or thalassaemia. This is complex and difficult and patients with these disorders have a poor long term prognosis. In severe cases of anaemia medical management may include blood transfusion of packed cells but only when the expected benefits outweigh the risks involved.

PHARMACOLOGY FOCUS

■ Iron deficiency anaemia is usually treated with ferrous sulphate 200 mg two to three times daily. Patients are usually advised to take with food as it can cause gastric upset and are warned that it will discolour the stool.

- Vitamin B_{12} deficiency is overcome with intramuscular injections of hydroxocobalamin, 1 mg three times per week for 2 weeks followed by one injection every 3 months.
- Folic acid deficiency can be treated with an oral course of folic acid 5 mg daily for 4 months.
- High doses of opioid analgesia may be necessary for the patient having a sickle cell crisis as this condition produces severe pain.

PRIORITIES FOR NURSING CARE

Anaemia is always a symptom of an underlying disorder and therefore nursing care needs to be tailored to the individual's needs.

- *Activity* needs to be carefully managed to match the reduced levels of oxygen that are available to the body tissues. Fatigue and breathlessness should be avoided but the patient should still be encouraged to be as active as possible. Activity tolerance should be assessed at regular intervals.
- The combination of reduced activity and oxygen supply to the skin increases the risk for pressure sore formation. Skin care is essential including creams and emollients to avoid the skin becoming dry and itchy.
- *Ulcers* of the oral mucosa and soreness of the tongue may occur in pernicious and iron deficiency anaemia. Oral care should include mouthwashes and the use of a soft toothbrush.
- *Falls* are possible because of dizziness and weakness; the patient should therefore be assessed for mobility and assisted as appropriate.
- *Pain* may be very severe in sickle cell disease owing to tissue ischaemia and in some other forms of anaemia as a result of vascular occlusion or marrow hyperplasia. Careful assessment of pain levels is important together with prompt action to relieve pain with medication.
- *Lack of concentration*, drowsiness or confusion are possible due to the diminished oxygen carrying capacity of the blood causing cerebral hypoxia. Therefore close observation of patients and reorientation may be necessary.

- *Diet* is a key part of long-term therapy. The nurse should be aware of the foods that are high in
  - Iron: red meat, eggs, green leafy vegetables, dried fruit, bread, fish, whole grain cereals.
  - Vitamin B$_{12}$: red meats, liver, eggs and dairy produce.
  - Folic acid: red meat, whole grain cereals, leafy vegetables, beans and dairy products.
  - Vitamin C: Citrus fruit and vegetables.
- *Health education* about diet and lifestyle are major parts of the long-term care plan for the patient. Before this can be fully effective the patient first has to understand the nature of their disorder. There is a great deal of health education work for the nurse to do, in conjunction with the dietician, in preparing the patient for discharge and to support the patient in the community thereafter.

LEUKAEMIA (P389)

PATHOLOGY: Key facts

Leukaemia is a term that covers a range of diseases involving haematopoietic cells. They are characterized by uncontrolled proliferation of immature blood cells and it is thought this arises from a single mutated early progenitor or stem cell. The immature abnormal cells overwhelm the red bone marrow and prevent the formation of normal red and white blood cells and platelets. Anaemia, reduced resistance to infection and bleeding disorders are therefore common problems. Leukaemias are classified according to how rapidly they progress (acute/chronic) and which type of leukocytes are the originators of the malignant cell division (myeloid/lymphoid). Leukaemia can affect all age groups and the disease can be fulminating and rapidly fatal or the person may live for many years with the disease. Exposure to ionizing radiation is one known environmental cause (demonstrated amongst survivors of the atom bombs dropped on Hiroshima and Nagasaki), and certain chemicals have also been implicated in causing the disease. However, in the majority of cases, the cause is still unknown.

WHAT TO LOOK OUT FOR

- *Acute leukaemia*
  - Tiredness, shortness of breath, recurrent infections and generally feeling unwell.
  - Bruising, nose bleeds, bleeding gums, very heavy menstrual bleeds.
  - In severe cases there may be septicaemia whilst internal haemorrhage can affect various systems causing, for example, brain damage or loss of sight (retinal bleed).
  - Acute myeloid leukaemia is most often seen in adults whilst acute lymphoblastic anaemia is most commonly a disease of childhood.
- *Chronic leukaemia*
  - Signs of anaemia such as fatigue and breathlessness.
  - Patients tend to be older than in acute leukaemia and with a more gradual onset. Some may not even be aware of symptoms, the illness only being detected when bloods are taken for some other reason.
  - Left-sided abdominal pain associated with an enlarged spleen.
  - The condition advances slowly at first but tends to accelerate the longer it remains undetected with the result that some patient may present in an acutely ill condition if they are only diagnosed late.

MEDICAL MANAGEMENT

Diagnosis is made from a detailed laboratory analysis of bone marrow aspirate which allows identification of the type of leukaemia present. Other investigations include full blood counts, biochemistry, clotting screen, chest radiograph and assessment of key organ function such as kidneys and liver. The patient's condition needs to be stabilized by administration of the appropriate blood products (concentrated red cells for anaemia, platelets for thrombocytopenic bleeding) and antibiotics to deal with any infection.

A central venous catheter needs to be inserted to allow for the administration of powerful cytotoxic drugs which will usually induce a rapid remission of the disease (p406). Unfortunately, these drugs will also cause anaemia and further bleeding disorder by their effect on erythrocytes and platelets so continual monitoring of blood parameters and further infusions of concentrated red cells and platelets are essential. While this intensive chemotherapy can deal effectively with the leukaemia and induce remission, these highly toxic drugs also have a wide range of adverse effects on the patient, who will require intensive support from all members of the care team. Male patients may be offered the opportunity to have sperm banked before chemotherapy as one of the many side effects will be destruction of fertility.

Maintenance therapy involves lower doses of cytotoxic drugs given on an outpatient basis. At this stage, some patients may be considered for allogenic bone marrow transplantation (from another person whose genetic make-up closely resembles the patient) or autologous stem cell transplantation (patient's own stem cells which have been collected before treatment with radio/chemotherapy). (See p395.)

FOCUS ON PHARMACOLOGY

The main emphasis is on the use of cytotoxic (cell-killing) drugs which work by disrupting cellular replication. As the malignant bone marrow cells are the most rapidly dividing, they are the ones most affected; however, all cells in the body which are undergoing cell division may be adversely affected. This gives rise to a range of side effects. Combinations of drugs are more effective than single drugs as each drug has a different mode of action thereby increasing cell death rates when used in combination with others. New types of drugs (immunotherapy) such as monoclonal antibodies and cytokines such as granulocyte colony stimulating factor have recently been introduced (p204). They enhance the body's own natural defence mechanisms and assist in the fight against cancers such as leukaemia whilst reducing side effects of the main cytotoxic drugs.

PRIORITIES FOR NURSING CARE

■ Rigorous infection control measures as chemotherapy leads to profound bone marrow failure and the risk of life-threatening infection.

- Care of the central venous line to ensure patency and minimize risk of introducing infection (p406).
- Fluid and nutritional support, including dietary supplements.
- Management of chemotherapy-induced symptoms such as nausea, vomiting, diarrhoea, mucositis (sore mouth and gums), anorexia, pain, pyrexia, hair loss, weight loss (radiotherapy produces similar problems, see p208).
- Assistance with all aspects of personal hygiene.
- Pressure area care.
- Psychological support for both patient and family.

MALIGNANT LYMPHOMAS (P398)

PATHOLOGY: Key facts

This term refers to a group of malignant diseases that affect lymphatic tisssue rather than the bone marrow. The most common form is Hodgkin's disease, while others are known simply as non-Hodgkin's lymphomas and usually involve the B and T lymphocytes. The lymph nodes and spleen become enlarged and proliferating cells may invade other organs and tissue. The cause of Hodgkin's disease remains unknown but it affects males more than females with peak incidence between 20 and 30 years of age, and after 50. The 5-year survival rate of Hodgkin's disease used to be only 20% in the 1960s, but is now 90% thanks to improved treatment.

WHAT TO LOOK OUT FOR

Hodgkin's Disease
- Gradual onset.
- Initially, painless enlargement of a set of lymph nodes (frequently cervical) followed by spread to other lymphoid and non-lymphoid tissue.
- Enlarging nodes cause pain (by pressure on nerve endings) and dysfunction of adjacent organs (e.g. enlarged mediastinal nodes cause a distressing cough, shortness of breath or difficulty swallowing).

■ In the later stages, anorexia, weight loss, fatigue, weakness and itching (pruritus).

Non-Hodgkin's Lymphoma

■ Gradual onset.
■ Painless enlargement of peripheral lymph nodes or a more generalized picture may present involving chest and abdomen.
■ Depending upon which areas are affected , the enlarging lymphatic tissues cause obstructive symptoms such as ascites, respiratory difficulty, lower limb oedema or intestinal obstruction.
■ Weight loss, fatigue, pyrexia.

MEDICAL MANAGEMENT

Investigations include full blood count, bone marrow aspiration and biopsy, liver function tests, chest radiography, immunoglobulin investigations. Other imaging techniques such as magnetic resonance imaging (MRI) scans may be used. Management depends upon accurate diagnosis and staging of the disease to measure its spread (p400). In both Hodgkin's and non-Hodgkin's disease, radiotherapy is used to treat early stage disease, either alone or in combination with chemotherapy. Chemotherapy is used for advanced disease (stage III or IV). The exact combinations of radiotherapy and cytotoxic drugs depends upon the stage of the disease and the patient's medical condition.

PHARMACOLOGY FOCUS

Cytotoxic drugs are usually given at 4-weekly intervals over six cycles for Hodgkin's disease. Frequently used drugs are chlormethine, vincristine, procarbazine and prednisolone. A common combination for non-Hodgkin's is cyclophosphamide, doxorubicin, vincristine and prednisolone.

PRIORITIES FOR NURSING CARE

Priorities will be similar to the patient undergoing treatment for leukaemia although much treatment is given on an outpatient basis.

- Prevention of infection, especially involving the central line used for chemotherapy.
- Care of side effects resulting from chemo/radiotherapy (see leukaemia, above).
- Psychological support and encouragement in view of the high survival rates and the fact that during remission the person can live a normal life.
- Sperm banking to preserve fertility for males should be discussed if appropriate.
- A good out-of-hours support service and close liaison with primary health care providers is essential given the number of patients managed at home.

TEN TOP TIPS

1. Observe infection control precautions at all times.
2. Handle gently due to risk of bleeding and bruising.
3. Monitor closely for signs of infection.
4. Be alert for signs of internal bleeding (haematurea, melaena, etc.).
5. Allow time and do not rush patients who may be very tired and fatigued.
6. Observe pressure areas closely and practise regular pressure care.
7. Mouth care is a high priority.
8. Offer continual psychological support for both patient and family.
9. Ensure anti-emetic drugs are given regularly to help combat side effects of chemo/radiotherapy.
10. Encourage frequent small amounts of food and drink as tolerated.

4

Caring for the patient with a disorder of the gastrointestinal system

Anatomy at a glance   51
Physiology you need to know   52
Neoplastic disease   54
Peptic ulceration   59
Inflammatory bowel disease   62
Ten top tips   65

ANATOMY AT A GLANCE

The main structures of the gut are shown in Figure 4.1.

The gut is basically a muscular tube which has a similar structure throughout its entire length consisting of four layers:

- The inner layer is the mucosa which in the stomach and small intestine contains specialized cells with secretory or absorptive functions.
- The submucosa binds the mucosa to the muscularis.
- The muscularis (muscle) layer is composed of two layers of involuntary smooth muscle from the mid oesophagus onwards, each layer arranged in a longitudinal and circular pattern. Exceptions to this general plan are the upper oseophagus, which consists of voluntary muscle to permit the conscious act of swallowing, and the stomach, which has a third oblique layer of involuntary muscle.
- The serosa, a serous membrane of connective tissue which below the diaphragm consists of the visceral peritoneum.

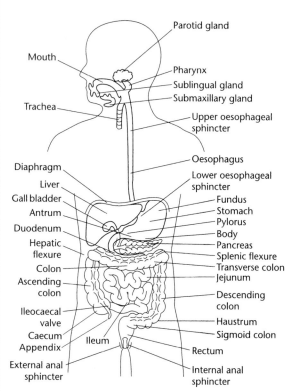

Figure 4.1 Structural divisions of the alimentary canal.

The gut terminates with the internal anal sphincter which connects the rectum to the anus (under involuntary control) and the external anal sphincter which connects the anus to the outside (under voluntary control).

PHYSIOLOGY YOU NEED TO KNOW

The gastrointestinal system supplies the body with the nutrients and fluids it needs to function, in an acceptable form. This is achieved by the ingestion, digestion and absorption of food and fluids.

The Stomach

Food is passed from the mouth via the oesophagus to the stomach where digestion begins. Ingested food and gastric secretions form a semi-liquid substance known as chyme which is continually churned and mixed by regular waves of muscle contraction in the stomach wall (peristalsis). The stomach mucosa contains many small gastric pits which are lined by:

- *Chief cells* which secrete pepsinogen. This is converted to pepsin when it comes into contact with hydrochloric acid. Pepsin is a powerful enzyme which breaks down proteins.
- *Parietal cells* which pump hydrogen and chloride ions into the stomach where they combine to form hydrochloric acid.
- *Mucus cells* which secrete mucus to protect the gastric mucosa from hydrochloric acid and pepsin.

Together with water, these components make up gastric juice which is highly acidic. This acid environment kills many bacteria and begins the breakdown of ingested food.

The Small Intestine

Digestion continues in the small intestine where enzymes (e.g. trypsin) continue the breakdown of proteins into amino acids, carbohydrates into glucose and other sugars (e.g. amylase) and fats into fatty acids and glycerol (lipase). Many of these enzymes are contained in intestinal juice secreted by cells in the intestinal wall and pancreatic juice. Bile secreted by the liver helps to emulsify fats in the duodenum, thereby facilitating fat digestion. Absorption takes place through many small projections on the small intestine wall called villi each of which in turn is covered by millions of minute hair-like projections called microvilli. The absorbed substances are carried away in the hepatic portal vein to the liver and then are made available to the rest of the body after a range of metabolic processes take place in the liver (first pass metabolism).

The Colon

The large intestine (colon) is predominantly the site of water and electrolyte absorption. A great deal of bacterial activity takes place in the colon but these bacteria are normally not pathogenic and help the body by synthesizing useful substances such as vitamin K (essential for the manufacture of prothrombin), folic acid and thiamine. Large quantities of mucus are also produced in the colon. Irritation of the colon wall increases mucus output and also causes the outpouring of water and electrolytes in an attempt to dilute and wash away the irritant. The result is diarrhoea.

NEOPLASTIC DISEASE

The gut is a major site of neoplastic disease. Three of the ten most common cancers in men affect the bowel, stomach and oesophagus whilst in women, cancer of the bowel is second only to cancer of the breast in incidence.

PATHOLOGY: Key facts

- *Oesophageal cancer* (p440) is increasing in frequency. It is more common in men, typically aged 50–70 and most commonly occurs in the lower third. The ability to swallow is progressively impaired and the growth spreads to involve surrounding organs such as the trachea, bronchi and stomach. The prognosis is poor with few patients surviving more than a year from diagnosis.

- *Stomach cancer* (p448) has the highest death rate in the age range 55–60 although the overall death rate has been falling in recent years. Predisposing factors are benign gastric ulceration, gastritis, *Helicobacter pylori* infection and pernicious anaemia. Gastric cancer invades adjacent organs and also spreads rapidly around the body as metastases via the lymphatic system.

- *Bowel cancer* (p477) most frequently occurs in the rectum. The sigmoid colon, caecum and ascending colon are the next most common sites. Cancers of the small bowel are very rare. Cancer of the colon is multifactorial in cause. A high-fat diet rich in red meat but poor in fruit and vegetables and lack of exercise are associated with an increased risk whilst some 20% of colorectal cancers have a genetic cause (e.g. familial polyposis) or a familial predisposition.

WHAT TO LOOK OUT FOR

- *Oesophageal cancer* Difficulty in swallowing (dysphagia) solids occurs first followed by problems with swallowing liquids. Discomfort and pain in the sub-sternal region may be accompanied by regurgitation. Loss of weight and strength develop as the person's food intake diminishes.

- *Stomach cancer* has an insidious onset, gradually belching, regurgitation, nausea and vomiting develop associated with a loss of appetite, weight and strength. Blood may appear in the vomitus or colouring the stool (melaena). Pain is a relatively late sign.

- *Bowel cancer* usually manifests itself by a change in regular bowel habit (alternating diarrhoea or constipation) and blood in the stool which may also be steaked with mucus. The person's overall health deteriorates as they feel tired and generally unwell, lose weight and develop anaemia. The person will often describe a feeling of incomplete evacuation when they defecate. Pain is again a late symptom and, generally speaking, the higher the cancer (e.g. in the caecum) the later the presentation as symptoms are not so apparent in the early stages.

MEDICAL MANAGEMENT

Oesophageal cancer is diagnosed by oesophagoscopy and/or barium swallow. Surgical intervention may be attempted in early cases to attempt to remove the tumour. In more advanced cases, the surgeon may only be able to introduce a feeding tube or stent to bypass the tumour and allow nutrition. Radiotherapy may also be offered to help reduce the size of the tumour.

Stomach cancer is diagnosed after endoscopy and biopsy, barium meal radiography and cytological studies of gastric juice. Computerized tomography may also be ordered to investigate the size and spread of the tumour in the abdomen and thorax. Surgery is the treatment of choice, the exact nature of the operation depending upon the tumour and its development. The lower oesophagus, omentum, spleen, pancreas or sections of the duodenum may also be involved in the surgery, depending upon the spread of the tumour. Radiotherapy and chemotherapy have so far not made any significant contribution to treatment of this cancer.

In *bowel cancer*, screening by faecal occult blood testing is being introduced as early detection greatly improves survival. Sigmoidoscopy or colonoscopy (and biopsy) coupled with barium enema investigations usually confirms the provisional diagnosis made from the history. Surgery to remove the tumour and a section of disease-free bowel either side is the treatment of choice. The two cut ends of the bowel are then surgically joined together (anastomosed). If the tumour is within a few centimetres of the anus, the rectum and anus are excised and a permanent colostomy formed. Radiotherapy and or chemotherapy may also be offered, particularly in advance of surgery, to shrink the size of the tumour.

PHARMACOLOGICAL FOCUS

Treatment of cancers of the gastrointestinal tract is primarily surgical, there are therefore no specific drugs unique to these disorders. Opioid analgesia is obviously important in the postoperative recovery phase for pain relief whilst in terminal illness, it plays a key role in palliative care.

PRIORITIES FOR NURSING CARE

■ *Oesophageal* cancer patients need:
  ● Nutritional support such as special diet and nutritional supplements. Food must be of a consistency that they can swallow.
  ● Fluid balance charting and assistance and encouragement with drinking to ensure hydration.
  ● Oral toilet and mouth care due to risk of regurgitation.
  ● Privacy, support and easily accessible vomit bowl if regurgitation is a problem.
  ● Psychological support to deal with altered body image (serious weight loss may occur) and the knowledge that they have a terminal disease.

- Pain control postoperatively and in advanced stages of the disease when pain becomes a problem.
- Full pre- and post-operative care if surgery is being undertaken.
- Encouragement with mobility and pressure area care as they may be at high risk of pressure sore development.
- Assistance with personal hygiene and comfort measures.

■ *Stomach* cancer patients need:

- Post-op care for the surgery undertaken (p454). This includes the following priorities:

    1. Care of nasogastric/nasointestinal or gastrostomy tube to ensure patency and security. This will prevent a build-up of secretions and other fluids at the site of surgery. Drainage should be charted accurately and regularly.
    2. Care of wound site.
    3. Careful removal of tube upon surgeon's instructions, usually once the patient can tolerate oral fluids.
    4. Frequent measurement of vital signs.
    5. Pain management. Patient-controlled analgesia (PCA) systems are very effective in patients that have had major abdominal surgery.
    6. Promotion of respiratory function. Breathing may be very painful and there may be thoracic drains left in situ, depending upon the surgical procedure carried out. There is a real risk of developing a serious postoperative chest infection, therefore deep breathing and coughing exercises are essential.
    7. Fluid and nutritional intake. Parenteral fluids are needed at first but will be phased out in favour of oral intake as bowel sounds return (indicating normal peristalsis in the gut). Accurate charting of fluid input and output is essential.
    8. Nutritional deficiencies need to be made up with dietary supplements and a carefully designed nutritional plan involving the dietician.
    9. Anaemia is a frequent problem because of chronic blood loss and poor preoperative diet. It may also

develop subsequently as a result of loss of intrinsic factor as the area of the stomach that normally secreted it, has been removed. Vitamin B_{12} injections may be needed for the rest of the person's life to prevent pernicious anaemia.

10. Alterations in diet and eating habits. The removal of a large part of the stomach means that the patient has to learn new eating habits to adapt to this major anatomical alteration. Frequent smaller meals, a well-balanced mix of essential foods to give the right number of calories and dietary constituents and regular weighing are essential to maintain health. Much patient education is therefore required both in hospital and in the community after discharge.

11. General post-op measures including oral toilet, care and assistance with personal hygiene, early mobility, psychological support and comfort measures.

● Long-term community support as they adapt to the changes referred to above (6, 7, 8).

● Ultimately they may need palliative care.

■ *Bowel* cancer patients will usually undergo surgery and need the following:

● Post-op care (p481):

1. Respiratory care, oxygen (prn) and deep breathing/coughing exercises.

2. Frequent measurements of vital signs.

3. Pain control, opioid analgesia via PCA and appropriate anti-emetic in short term. Ensure adequate analgesia medium/long term also.

4. Care of wound site including colostomy if necessary.

5. Fluid balance charting, care of IVI until discontinued, encouragement with oral fluids.

6. Gradual increase in oral intake of fluids and then semi-solids and solid foods as bowel sounds return.

7. Care of urinary catheter and accurate charting of urine output after catheter is removed.

8. Monitor bowel movements, lactulose may be considered if there has been no movement 5 days post-op.

9. Encourage mobility and use of anti-embolism stockings to avoid DVT.

10. Other general post-op care such as assistance with personal hygiene, regular monitoring of pressure areas and comfort measures.

11. Psychological support to assist patient to work through the stress of major surgery for a life-threatening condition and the changes in body image that have occurred.

12. Discharge plan involving community nursing staff and patient education concerning important topics such as long-term recovery from surgery, diet, risk of recurrence of cancer, warning signs to look out for, long-term care of colostomy if one has been formed and general lifestyle advice.

PEPTIC ULCERATION (P444)

PATHOLOGY: Key facts

Hydrochloric acid and the enzyme pepsin, both key components of gastric juice, are capable of causing inflammation and ulceration of the oesophagus, stomach and duodenum. This normally does not happen:

- In the oesophagus because gastric juice is kept within the stomach by the cardiac sphincter.
- In the stomach because the large quantity of mucus secreted by the mucus cells forms a protective barrier several millimetres thick over the gastric mucosa.
- In the duodenum because strongly alkaline substances are added to chyme to neutralize its acidity (e.g. bile, pancreatic juice and intestinal secretions).
- Because a normal healthy mucosa can rapidly regenerate new cells if any are destroyed.

If any factor interferes with these defensive mechanisms, inflammation and ulceration occur and the bacterium *H. pylori* is the main factor responsible for such disturbances and therefore peptic ulceration or malignancy. Other factors implicated in causing inflammation and ulceration are:

- Stress associated with severe illness and major trauma.
- Genetic predisposition.
- Certain drugs such as corticosteroids and the non-steroidal anti-inflammatory drugs (NSAIDs) of which aspirin and ibuprofen are the most common.
- Bile reflux into the stomach due to an incompetent pyloric sphincter.
- Histamine promotes acid secretion.
- Failure of the cardiac sphincter leads to gastro-oesophageal reflux and is usually associated with hiatus hernia (protrusion of part of the stomach into the thorax via a weakness in the diaphragm where the oesophagus passes through). Oesophageal ulceration results.
- Smoking.
- Endocrine disorders can lead to gastric hypersecretion (e.g. Zollinger–Ellison syndrome where a tumour of the pancreatic islets of Langerhans causes over-production of the hormone gastrin).
- Chronic gastritis (inflammation) predisposes to gastric ulceration or gastric cancer.

WHAT TO LOOK OUT FOR

- *Oesophagitis (inflammation of the oesophagus)* causes the familiar symptom of heartburn. Substernal pain, intolerance of spicy foods and dysphagia may also be present.
- *Chronic gastritis (inflammation of the gastric mucosa)* produces various vague symptoms such as 'heartburn', 'indigestion' a feeling of fullness and discomfort, nausea and loss of appetite.
- *Peptic ulceration* produces epigastric pain described as gnawing or gripping in nature. It is usually associated consistently with eating, with gastric ulcers producing pain within an hour of eating whilst duodenal ulcers typically produce pain 2–4 hours after a meal. The patient may be woken during the night by the pain, which may be confused with cardiac pain. Should a peptic ulcer erode through a blood vessel, severe bleeding occurs with haematemesis (vomiting blood), shock and collapse. The patient has a rigid abdomen and is in severe pain. This is a surgical emergency with potentially life-threatening

consequences. Complete perforation of the stomach or duodenal wall is equally serious as gut contents spill out into the abdominal cavity causing peritonitis.

MEDICAL MANAGEMENT

Careful endoscopic investigation is needed to confirm the diagnosis. The presence of *H. pylori* may be confirmed by use of a breath test kit or by serology. Treatment is directed towards healing the ulcer, relieving symptoms, preventing complications and avoiding a recurrence. Drug therapy (see below) and lifestyle/dietary modifications form the main approach to treatment. Surgery is occasionally necessary if the ulcer proves intractable; a subtotal gastrectomy is performed to remove the ulcer-bearing area of the stomach. Vagotomy is a surgical procedure sometimes combined with subtotal gastrectomy. It involves dividing the vagus nerve thereby reducing gastric secretion. In the event of a perforation or bleed, emergency surgery may be needed to repair the damaged area.

PHARMACOLOGY FOCUS

The following are the main drugs used in the management of peptic ulceration:

■ H_2-receptor antagonists. This group of drugs blocks histamine receptor sites (known as H_2 receptors), thereby reducing hydrochloric acid secretion by the parietal cells. Examples are cimetidine and ranitidine.
■ Proton pump inhibitors interfere with the ability of parietal cells to produce hydrochloric acid, e.g. omeprazole.
■ Antibiotic regimens to eradicate *H. pylori* infection are added to a proton pump inhibitor in what is known as 'triple therapy'. A typical and common regime consists of a 2-week course of omeprazole (20 mg×2/day), clarithromycin (500 mg×2/day) and amoxicillin (1 g×2/day).
■ Antacids (typically based on aluminium or magnesium compounds) can relieve symptoms between meals and are helpful in less serious cases. Taken in large doses,

however, they can cause significant electrolyte and other physiological disturbances.

■ Alginates (e.g. Gaviscon) are useful for mild to moderate gastro-oesophageal reflux disease. They form a 'raft' over stomach contents and so inhibit reflux into the oesophagus.

PRIORITIES FOR NURSING CARE

The vast majority of patients are managed in primary care. Practice nurses and nurse practitioners play a key role in health education about lifestyle modification (diet, eating habits, smoking cessation, alcohol reduction, stress management) and the correct use of drugs, especially over-the-counter medication such as the H_2-receptor antagonists and antacids. They are also responsible for ensuring that patients are investigated should symptoms persist or worsen.

Admission usually only occurs if there is an acute exacerbation and nursing care will focus on monitoring vital signs, checking for complications such as haemorrhage, general supportive measures, ensuring correct medication is administered and pain relief.

INFLAMMATORY BOWEL DISEASE (P468)

PATHOLOGY: Key facts

The two main conditions are Crohn's disease and ulcerative colitis. They predominantly affect young adults and are most common in the developed world. These are separate conditions. Their cause is not clear although aetiology is likely to be multifactorial and there is a genetic predisposition. The psychological disturbance associated with these diseases is a consequence of the disorder rather than a cause.

■ *Crohn's disease* can affect any part of the intestine. Patches of granulomatous inflammation and ulceration develop which can erode through the full thickness of the intestinal wall leading to perforation of the bowel.

■ *Ulcerative colitis* is confined to the colon and consists of severe inflammation and ulceration of the mucosa.

WHAT TO LOOK OUT FOR

Ulcerative Colitis

The severity of the disorder may vary but the following are found in more-severe cases.

■ Diarrhoea consisting of watery stools which may contain blood, mucus and pus and which are passed up to 20 times per day.
■ Urgency and cramping abdominal pains accompany the diarrhoea.
■ Reduced food intake and weight loss.
■ Fatigue and malaise.
■ Fever and dehydration.

Crohn's Disease

Generally, the person has chronic but mild symptoms with occasional more severe acute episodes. In acute exacerbations the person has:

■ Abdominal pain accompanied by a sensation of cramping and tenderness.
■ Flatulence, nausea and diarrhoea, though this is less severe than ulcerative colitis.
■ Anorexia and malaise.
■ Abscesses and/or a fistula may form leading to fever and the risk of adhesions and partial bowel obstruction.

MEDICAL MANAGEMENT

Careful investigation is necessary to arrive at a diagnosis. This involves:

■ Stool cultures to eliminate gastroenteritis as a cause of the patients symptoms.
■ Sigmoidoscopy allows direct examination of the rectum and sigmoid colon.
■ Colonoscopy allows examination of the entire colon.
■ Radiological investigations include barium studies which outline the lumen of the intestine with barium sulphate (barium enema).

Once a diagnosis has been made drug therapy forms the basis of medical treatment although complications such as a bowel obstruction may lead to surgical intervention in cases of Crohn's disease. If ulcerative colitis proves intractable and severely disabling, the patient may require the surgical removal of the entire colon and rectum with the formation of an ileostomy where the terminal ileum is brought to the abdominal wall for purposes of emptying.

PHARMACOLOGY FOCUS

The main drugs used are anti-inflammatory agents, immunosuppressants and antibiotics.

- *Corticosteroids* have both an anti-inflammatory and immunosuppressant effect and may be given via the oral, intravenous or rectal routes. The patient should be closely monitored after discharge for the long-term side effects of steroid therapy.
- *Sulfasalazine* has an anti-infective and anti-inflammatory action. A minimum fluid intake of 2500 mL/day is necessary to avoid the formation of sulfonamide crystals in the kidneys and subsequent renal damage.
- *Antibiotics* such as metronidazole are necessary if an infected fistula or abscess forms.
- *Antidiarrhoeal* agents may also be prescribed on a symptomatic basis.

Additionally, immunosupressive therapy (azathioprine) may be used in patients who cannot tolerate steroids and recently monoclonal antibody treatment (infliximab) has been introduced for those that are severely ill.

PRIORITIES FOR NURSING CARE

Acute Episodes Requiring Admission

- Parenteral nutrition is frequently needed to allow the bowel to recover and to improve the patient's nutritional status. A central vein is usually cannulated to allow solutions of protein, glucose, lipids, electrolytes, etc., to be administered while an automatic pump regulates the rate of flow. Strict asepsis is necessary at all times because of the major infection risk posed by this procedure.

- Meticulous mouth care is essential as the patient is unable to eat and often cannot drink either.
- Vital signs must be monitored frequently to detect early signs of infection or other complications.
- Daily weight and fluid balance charting.
- Pressure care together with the full regime of care needed for a patient who has very limited mobility to avoid complications such as deep vein thrombosis (DVT).
- Assistance with personal hygiene.
- Drug therapy including pain relief as required.
- Psychological support is essential as the patient will probably have had their personal life already disrupted by this stressful and chronic condition. Disturbance in body image and self esteem are common.

Preparation for Discharge and Care at Home

A great deal of patient education is needed to help the person and their family live with this long-term condition. Key areas include:

- Explanation of the actual disease process and indicators of deterioration such as significant weight loss, change in bowel habit.
- Correct dosage and timing of medication together with side effects.
- Encouragement to try and live as normal a life as possible when feeling well.
- Offer of counselling to help the person deal with the psychological impact of the disorder.
- Discussion about the impact of the disorder on their sex life.
- Referral to a self-help group.

TEN TOP TIPS

1. Pain frequently accompanies these conditions so monitor regularly and be sure to give analgesia as required.
2. Check stools carefully and accurately record any unusual features.

3. Vomiting is a distressing symptom, be prepared with bowls, mouthwash, tissues and again note the quantity and type of vomitus.
4. Encourage the patient to talk about their fears; the possibility of cancer is a major worry for many.
5. Invasive investigations are common so ensure that the patient has a full explanation of what to expect.
6. Monitor vital signs closely if the patient is an acute admission as shock and sepsis associated with a perforation can develop rapidly.
7. Take opportunities to discuss the importance of a high-fibre diet as a means of avoiding constipation.
8. Explore people's understanding of what constitutes a healthy diet and offer appropriate health education.
9. Respect the dietary preferences of various cultures and religions.
10. Check that patient is actually eating the food given to them on the ward.

5

Caring for the patient with a disorder of the liver, biliary tract and exocrine pancreas

Anatomy at a glance   67
Physiology you need to know   68
Cirrhosis of the liver   69
Hepatitis   73
Jaundice   76
Pancreatitis   78
Cholelithiasis (gall stones)   82
Ten top tips   83

ANATOMY AT A GLANCE

These closely associated structures are located in the upper abdominal cavity immediately below the diaphragm (Figure 5.1). The liver is a large organ weighing approximately 1.4 kg and is situated in the upper right portion of the abdomen. The gall bladder is much smaller (7–10 cm in length) and is located under the liver. Bile is passed from the liver to the gall bladder via the left and right hepatic ducts and subsequently into the duodenum via the bile duct. The pancreas lies across the upper abdomen being 12–15 cm long but only 2.5 cm thick. The head of the pancreas is located by the curve of the duodenum and the body and tail lie to the left of the head. Pancreatic secretions drain via the pancreatic duct into the duodenum. Normally, the pancreatic duct and bile duct enter the duodenum together as a common duct known as the ampulla of Vater.

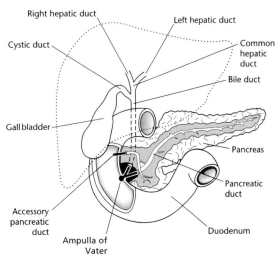

Figure 5.1 The pancreas and associated anatomy.

PHYSIOLOGY YOU NEED TO KNOW

■ *The liver* has many vital functions and is metabolically extremely active. Key functions of the liver include:

● Formation of bilirubin from the haem of degraded old red blood cells which is then secreted into bile and passed to the duodenum to assist digestion of fats by emulsification of lipids.

● Synthesis of bile salts which also assist in digestion of fats.

● Processing of drugs and hormones.

● Phagocytosis of aged red and white blood cells plus some bacteria is carried out by Kupffer cells.

● Storage of vitamins such as A, B_{12}, D, E and K plus minerals such as iron.

● Maintenance of blood glucose levels by converting glucose to glycogen and triglycerides for storage when blood glucose levels are high. When blood glucose levels are low, stored glycogen is broken down into glucose and released into the bloodstream. Amino acids and lactose can also be converted to glucose.

- Protein metabolism. Amino acids have the amino group removed from them by liver cells so they can be used for adenosine triphosphate (ATP) production. ATP is a key energy source for body cells. This deamination forms ammonia which is converted into the less harmful substance urea which is excreted in urine.
- Lipid metabolism. This includes synthesizing cholesterol and using it to make bile salts and breaking down fatty acids to make ATP.
- Synthesis of the active form of vitamin D along with the skin and kidneys.

■ *The gall bladder.* The liver secretes up to 1 L per day of strongly alkaline bile. It is stored and concentrated by a factor of up to 10 in the gall bladder before excretion into the small intestine, particularly to help digest the fatty portion of a meal.

■ *The exocrine pancreas* constitutes 99% of this organ, the remaining 1% is the endocrine portion concerned with the secretion of hormones such as insulin and glucagon. The exocrine pancreas secretes pancreatic juice which contains a range of digestive enzymes needed in the small intestine. These include:

- Amylase to digest carbohydrate.
- Several protein-digesting enzymes such as the inactive enzyme tripsinogen which is converted to active tripsin when it encounters enterokinase within the small intestine.
- Lipase which digests triglycerides.

CIRRHOSIS OF THE LIVER (P509)

PATHOLOGY: Key facts

Chronic and diffuse degeneration of the liver associated with the formation of scar tissue characterizes cirrhosis. The liver becomes congested, function deteriorates and portal hypertension ensues. Portal hypertension is associated with the development of ascites – the accumulation of large quantities of fluid in the abdomen due to disruption of the normal balance of pressures in the capillary bed impairing the return of fluid to the venous capillaries. The most likely cause is alcohol abuse although many alcoholics do not develop cirrhosis. Cirrhotic changes can also occur after chronic hepatitis, obstruction of bile flow (e.g. due to gallstones) or in response to autoimmune processes.

WHAT TO LOOK OUT FOR

Onset is slow and insidious as the liver has considerable spare capacity. Early signs of liver dysfunction include:

- Digestive disturbances and nausea.
- Anorexia.
- Weight loss.
- Flatulence.
- Pruritus or itching of the skin.

Later signs include:

- Jaundice.
- Dependent oedema.
- Anaemia.
- Increased abdominal girth due to ascites.
- Spider angiomas.

In advanced cases, the person will have an enlarged spleen, neurological signs possibly leading to a hepatic coma and bleeding from oesophageal varices (oesophageal veins with the characteristic changes of varicose veins).

MEDICAL MANAGEMENT

Liver function tests (LFT) measure the levels of key enzymes and are important in determining the severity of the disease in addition to the history and physical signs found upon examination. Interpretation of LFT results is complex, but elevated aminotransferases generally indicates liver cell damage. Blood tests are also important as an extended prothrombin time indicates clotting disorder. This is significant, as the liver synthesizes many of the blood coagulation factors.

Once the diagnosis is confirmed, alcohol intake must be eliminated, if that is the cause, to prevent further damage. There is no cure for cirrhosis although liver transplant may be offered if the person is willing to give up drinking. Medical management is usually symptomatic involving fluid restrictions and the cautious use of diuretics to reduce ascites. If the volume of ascites is interfering with respiration, paracentesis is performed using a sterile cannula to tap off the excess fluid from the peritoneal cavity.

PHARMACOLOGY FOCUS

There are no specific drug therapies that treat cirrhosis. Hepatic neurological disorder is caused by the failure of the liver to metabolize and detoxify nitrogenous substances, therefore part of the treatment involves reducing the levels of these substances in the body. As one of the main functions of the liver is to metabolize drugs and hormones, all medication should be carefully reviewed as normally therapeutic doses could quickly become toxic. Drugs which are normally inactivated in the liver such as paracetamol, diazepam, oral contraceptives and opiates are excluded.

PRIORITIES FOR NURSING CARE

- Careful observation of the patient is essential for the following:
  - Vital signs.
  - Any bleeding tendencies (bruising, melaena).
  - Fluid balance and nutritional intake.
  - Daily weights.
  - Level of consciousness for signs of confusion, drowsiness or alcohol withdrawal symptoms.
  - Evidence of jaundice.
- Itching can be a major problem so apply anti-pruritic lotions and moisturisers, keep skin cool and change bedding daily. Assist with personal hygiene and keep nails short.
- Assist with and encourage nutrition in accordance with dietician's orders. Typically, this will involve a high-calorie (2500–3000 kcal/day) high-carbohydrate diet with vitamin supplements. Protein content may be limited or

excluded completely depending upon the patient's condition due to the toxic effects of accumulating nitrogenous waste substances which the liver is unable to metabolize.

- Encourage upright position to assist breathing if ascites is a problem.
- Assist with mobility and provide pressure area care.
- The problem of alcohol intake will have to be discussed if this is thought to be the cause of the problem (p.913). Box 5.1 reveals some key facts about alcohol intake, while Box 5.2 shows recommended daily intake limits. A useful tool which assesses whether a patient has an alcohol problem is shown in Box 5.3. If the patient answers yes to more than one of these questions, this indicates a likely problem. This can be used in primary care settings as well as in a hospital.
- Patient education is crucial as there is no medical cure for cirrhosis, the patient has to learn to live with the disease and adapt their lifestyle accordingly to minimize its impact. Alcohol consumption is clearly contraindicated,

---

Box 5.1 Alcohol consumption in the UK

- In England in 2002, nearly two-fifths (37%) of men drank more than 4 units of alcohol in one day in the previous week; around one-fifth of women (22%) drank more than three units of alcohol in one day in the previous week.
- In England in 2002, 21% of men had drunk more than 8 units of alcohol in a day, at least once in the previous week, compared with 9% of women.
- In 2002, mean weekly alcohol consumption in England was 17 units for men and 7.6 units for women.
- In England in 2002, 27% of men and 17% of women aged 16 years and over were drinking more than 21 and 14 units a week, respectively. Drinking at these levels amongst men has remained stable at about 27% since 1992; that of women has risen from about 12%.
- More than one-quarter (27%) of pupils aged 11–15 years drank in the previous week in 2003 in England, compared with one-fifth (20%) in 1988.

From Department of Health (2004) Statistics on alcohol: England, 2004. Online. Available: www.dh.gov.uk/PublicationsAndStatistics/StatisticalWorkAreas

Box 5.2 Recommended daily alcohol intake limits

Men: 3–4 units
Women: 2–3 units

After an episode of drunkenness, alcohol should be avoided for at least 48 hrs to allow the body to recover

Department of Health (2006) Alcohol and Health. Online. Available: www.dh.gov.uk/PolicyAndGuidance/ HealthAndSocialCareTopics/AlcoholMisuse [Accessed 08.04.2006]

Box 5.3 The CAGE alcohol screen (p.929)

If the patient answers yes to any of these questions, they may have a problem

Cut down	Have you felt that you should cut down or stop drinking?
Annoyed	Have people annoyed you when they've told you that you should cut down or stop drinking?
Guilt	Have you ever felt guilty about how much you want to drink?
Eye-opener	Do you wake up in the morning wanting to have an alcoholic eye-opener drink?

From Gorman, M (1997) Treating acute alcohol withdrawal. *American Journal of Nursing* 97(1): 22–23.

however, some patients may be unable or unwilling to abstain leading to major health problems which may be compounded by related social problems such as family break up, unemployment and homelessness.

HEPATITIS (P506)

PATHOLOGY: Key facts

Hepatitis is a term used to describe inflammation of the liver. Hepatocytes (liver cells) are severely damaged and often die, resulting in potentially serious health problems. As the hepatocytes become inflamed, swelling and congestion occurs within the liver which interferes with the drainage of bile

Box 5.4 Summary of the different types of viral hepatitis

Type	Transmission	Characteristics
Hepatitis A	Faecal–oral route, associated with poor hygiene, contaminated food/water	Acute short-term illness, person does not become a carrier; children, young adults commonly infected
Hepatitis B	Injection of infected blood, blood products or sexually transmitted	Slow onset, chronic disease Most common in adults Person remains infective
Hepatitis C	Infected blood or blood products Low risk for sexual transmission	Mild disease, but up to 70% of patients develop chronic liver disease 85% of infected persons are unaware of their infection
Hepatitis D	Requires presence of hepatitis B for transmission to occur	Very rare in northern Europe
Hepatitis E	Enteric route	Only found in Asia

leading to obstructive jaundice. Long term, the disease may lead to fibrosis of the liver and cirrhosis. The main causes are viral or as a result of an autoimmune process often associated with alcohol, environmental toxins or drugs such as isoniazid or rifampicin. The disease may be acute or chronic.

WHAT TO LOOK OUT FOR

■ Onset is usually insidious with non-specific symptoms such as headaches, fatigue, appetite loss, nausea, vomiting, intermittent aches and pains in the joints.

- Several days later abdominal pain develops, particularly tenderness over the liver in the upper right quadrant.
- Jaundice is likely to develop with the characteristic dark urine and pale stools.
- Bleeding problems such as melaena, purpura (bruising) develop because of altered production and destruction of blood components necessary for normal clotting.
- Pruritus associated with the jaundice (accumulation of bile salts in the skin causes itching).

The severity of the disease varies considerably between individuals and many people make a complete recovery without long-term problems.

MEDICAL MANAGEMENT

Various blood tests are carried out to identify the type of virus responsible by looking for viral antibodies and antigens. Liver function tests check for raised enzymes such as alanine aminotransferase (ALT) and aspartate aminotransferase (AST), which indicate damaged liver cells. A liver biopsy is required to obtain a sample of liver tissue to check for fibrosis and cirrhosis.

There is no specific treatment for hepatitis, whatever the cause, other than general supportive measures. In advanced cases with serious liver damage, the patient may be considered for a liver transplant.

PHARMACOLOGY FOCUS

The emphasis is on prevention. Contacts of people with hepatitis A may be given protection by an injection of human immune serum globulin. Hepatitis B immune globulin is available for those who have been exposed through needle-stick injury or some other accident. Active immunization against hepatitis B is available for nurses and other health care staff, and involves a course of three injections with follow-up boosters.

Patients with chronic hepatitis B may be helped by the administration of interferon-α but this is expensive and still the subject of much debate as to its effectiveness.

PRIORITIES FOR NURSING CARE

- *Rest.* Bed rest, especially for young people acutely ill with hepatitis A, is needed to help the patient through an acute episode. If the patient is at home, rest is still advised and recovery monitored by checking liver function test results.

- *Medication.* The liver has a very important role in the metabolism of many drugs. The patient therefore should be advised against taking any drugs which have not been medically prescribed. A thorough review of medication should be carried out and careful observation maintained for any side effects from whatever drugs the patient remains on.

- *Nutrition and fluids.* Fluid intake of 3000 mL/day is needed to cope with the dehydrating effects of fever and to help promote urinary excretion of serum bilirubin. A high-calorie diet (3000 kcal/day) is also needed to help repair liver tissue but it should be low in fat content due to difficulties in fat digestion caused by the obstructive jaundice. No alcohol should be drunk for at least six months.

- *Skin care.* Jaundice makes the skin very itchy. Emollients in bathwater help, together with keeping skin cool and nails short.

- *Infection control.* Universal and body substance precautions are necessary as all patients with viral hepatitis are potentially infective. Always take great care with sharps to avoid the risk of needlestick injury. Lifestyle advice about the dangers of sharing needles with IV drug users should be offered. A major concern is the transmission of type C, especially through poorly run tattoo parlours, whilst the protective value of condom use should be stressed to homosexual patients to avoid type B infection

JAUNDICE (P502)

PATHOLOGY: Key facts

Jaundice is actually a sign of an underlying disorder rather than a disease in its own right. It is caused by an accumulation of excess bilirubin in the blood, which in turn causes the skin, mucous membranes and sclerae to have a yellowish colour. The main causes are:

- *Haemolytic* associated with excess breakdown of red blood cells and therefore destruction of haemoglobin and formation of bilirubin.
- *Hepatocellular* caused by damage to the liver cells as in hepatitis. The diseased hepatocytes are unable to take up the naturally formed bilirubin.
- *Obstructive* which may be either intrahepatic (e.g. cirrhosis) or extrahepatic (e.g. carcinoma of the head of the pancreas or impacted gall stones within the common hepatic duct). In either case, there is obstruction to the normal flow of bile from the liver into the duodenum.

WHAT TO LOOK OUT FOR

The yellow coloration of jaundice may not initially be obvious in the skin but is readily seen in the sclerae. This is particularly important in assessing people from a non-European ethnic background. The urine becomes dark due to the presence of bilirubin, which will show up on testing with a dipstick. Faeces are pale due to the absence of bile in the intestine in obstructive and hepatocellular jaundice.

The patient presents with an itchy skin (pruritus), and bruising may be apparent due to bleeding abnormalities, which develop secondary to liver disease owing to inadequate production of prothrombin and other blood clotting factors. Other common symptoms include:

- Loss of appetite and weight loss.
- Fatigue and weakness.
- Nausea and vomiting.
- Flatulence.
- Dull ache and tenderness in the liver region (right upper quadrant of abdomen).
- Low-grade fever may also be present.

MEDICAL MANAGEMENT

Medical staff will be attempting to diagnose the underlying cause and manage that disorder. Remember that jaundice is only a sign of something else.

PHARMACOLOGY FOCUS

This depends upon the underlying cause; however, it is wise to assume that any jaundiced patient may have significant liver disease which has serious implications for their medication, as most drugs are metabolized in the liver.

PRIORITIES FOR NURSING CARE

Jaundice produces a major change in a person's appearance and is therefore likely to affect self concept. Support and encouragement is needed together with the opportunity to talk about feelings. The person may have assumed that jaundice is such a serious sign they are likely to die. They may also assume that only 'drug addicts' get jaundice and hepatitis. Such issues need to be tactfully explored and misconceptions clarified.

PANCREATITIS (P519)

PATHOLOGY: Key facts

The term pancreatitis refers to inflammation of the pancreas which can be acute or chronic.

Acute Pancreatitis

This is caused when the proteinases and lipases (enzymes) secreted by the exocrine pancreas as part of the pancreatic juice, become activated within the pancreas rather than in the duodenum as happens normally. The result is that effectively the pancreas digests itself (autodigestion), with subsequent destruction of large areas of the pancreas and surrounding tissue. In severe cases, internal bleeding into the peritoneal cavity occurs along with peritonitis, paralytic ileus, severe pain and shock. Ultimately, this may become a life-threatening condition.

The trigger for this chain of events is usually a blockage in the flow of pancreatic juices within the duct system. A gallstone that has found its way through the sphincter of Oddi is the most likely cause; this causes a reflux of bile into the pancreas, which in turn activates the normally inert pancreatic enzymes within the pancreas itself. The overall mortality rate for acute pancreatitis is 10%, and if there is widespread cell destruction (necrotizing pancreatitis) this approaches 50%, indicating the severity of this condition.

Chronic Pancreatitis

This usually develops insidiously, and is associated with alcohol abuse, although it may occur secondary to an acute episode of pancreatitis. There is progressive fibrosis of the pancreas, and the effects upon the patient are proportional to the amount of healthy pancreatic tissue lost.

WHAT TO LOOK OUT FOR

Acute pancreatitis is characterized by a sudden and severe onset of symptoms. The person experiences severe abdominal pain, which is described as boring through to the back. Peritonitis (inflammation of the peritoneum) produces the classic picture of a rigid, distended abdomen (the person cannot bend). The patient will be severely distressed and quickly develop the signs of shock as blood pressure falls and pulse and breathing rates climb. Nausea and vomiting are common. Destruction of the islets of Langerhans can complicate the picture further by leading to hyperglycaemia and glucosuria. Inflammation and swelling of the head of the pancreas can lead to obstruction of the common bile duct and obstructive jaundice. Failure to absorb vitamin K leads to bleeding disorders.

The person with chronic pancreatitis experiences recurring episodes of abdominal pain around the right upper quadrant. Loss of appetite, nausea, flatulence and constipation also commonly occur. Eventually the pain may be unrelenting. Episodes are brought on by eating a large fatty meal or drinking alcohol. The loss of pancreatic enzymes leads to decreased efficiency of digestion, leading to weight loss and steatorrhoea (bulky, fatty and offensive stools). Diabetes mellitus may develop as the islets of Langerhans are progressively destroyed.

MEDICAL MANAGEMENT

Immediate priorities are to provide effective pain relief and resuscitate the patient. A central venous line and urinary catheter will be placed to facilitate management. Diagnosis depends upon finding raised serum amylase or lipase concentrations and ultrasound views showing swelling of the pancreas. Medical treatment is directed towards managing the various physiological disturbances that occur as a result of the condition such as hypovolaemic shock, hyperglycaemia, paralytic ileus and obstructive jaundice. If there is widespread destruction of the pancreas or evidence of abscess formation, surgical debridement of the diseased pancreas is undertaken together with drainage of the surrounding area.

The key to managing chronic pancreatitis is to persuade the patient to abstain totally from alcohol. This is, however, very difficult as the person is usually a heavy drinker with an alcohol-dependency problem. If they are abstemious and pain persists, they may be offered endoscopic therapy aimed at dilating or stenting the main pancreatic duct to promote drainage of pancreatic juices. Surgical intervention to resect part of the pancreas may also be considered. Oral pancreatic enzyme substitutes will reduce pancreatic activity and may help reduce pain.

PHARMACOLOGICAL FOCUS

Acute Pancreatitis

The following key medications will be required:

- Opioid analgesia for pain relief (pethidine also relaxes smooth muscle).
- IV saline or colloids to resuscitate the patient and then maintenance IV hydration.
- Insulin to combat hyperglycaemia.
- Parenteral nutrition will be needed to overcome the severe catabolic state that the patient usually develops.

Chronic Pancreatitis

- Long-term analgesia. Non-steroidal anti-inflammatory drugs (NSAIDs) should be the first line of management although opioids may have to be used if pain proves severe and unrelieved by NSAIDs. The long-term chronic nature of chronic pancreatitis has significant implications for the use of opioids as tolerance may develop leading to larger and larger doses being required.

- Prepared pancreatic extract (pancreatin) compensates for the loss of pancreatic enzymes. It is given orally, but is inactivated by gastric acid, and therefore must be taken with food. Ranitidine may be taken an hour before the pancreatin to reduce gastric acid secretion. The drug is also inactivated by heat so should not be mixed with hot foods. Dosage is adjusted to each individual patient depending upon the size, number and consistency of stools to produce the best results. Pancreatin is of porcine origin, therefore the religious beliefs of patients should be considered before therapy begins.
- Vitamin supplements such as A, D, K, folic acid and B_{12} may be required.

PRIORITIES FOR NURSING CARE

Acute Pancreatitis
- Analgesia and effective pain relief.
- Frequent observations of vital signs.
- Oxygen therapy if shocked.
- Care of IVI and urinary catheter with accurate fluid balance.
- Total parenteral nutrition.
- Pressure area care.
- Care of nasogastric tube.
- Monitor blood glucose levels and keep within normal range by insulin therapy.
- Assistance with personal hygiene.
- Early mobilization.
- Psychological support.
- Teaching about long-term care and lifestyle issues such as alcohol intake aimed at preventing the development of chronic pancreatitis.

Chronic Pancreatitis
- Education and assistance with alcohol withdrawal.
- Lifestyle advice and education.
- Information about analgesia.
- Teaching about use of pancreatin and adjusting dosage to produce best results in terms of optimising health, weight and stool formation (reducing steatorrhoea).
- Low-fat diet will assist with preventing steatorrhoea.

- Patient teaching about hyperglycaemia and insulin if required.
- Long-term vitamin supplements.

CHOLELITHIASIS (GALL STONES) (P517)

PATHOLOGY: Key facts

Cholelithiasis refers to the presence of stones (usually made up of cholesterol or bile pigments) in the gall bladder. They may produce little or no symptoms in some people, mild indigestion-like symptoms in others (associated with fatty foods) or severe pain known as biliary colic. There is much debate concerning the factors that cause stones to form. Cholesterol stones are most likely to form in people whose livers produce bile that has an excess of cholesterol (lithogenic bile), and where there are factors that can initiate the precipitation of biliary cholesterol into solid stones.

Stones can cause inflammation of the gall bladder (cholecystitis) or obstruct the flow of bile within the liver, impairing the function of that organ. An impacted stone in the common bile duct causes severe biliary colic and obstructive jaundice, as it blocks the free drainage of bile into the duodenum.

WHAT TO LOOK OUT FOR

Acute cholecystitis (inflammation of the gall bladder) produces pain in the right upper quadrant of the abdomen or the mid-epigastric region. Nausea, vomiting and fever are common. The patient may have a previous history suggesting that fatty foods induce indigestion.

Signs of jaundice are apparent if the stone is blocking the common bile duct.

MEDICAL MANAGEMENT

Investigations usually involve a procedure known as endoscopic retrograde cholangiopancreatography (ERCP). An endoscope is passed via the duodenum and ampulla of Vater into the bile and pancreatic ducts. A contrast medium may be injected to assist radiographic investigation during ERCP.

Acute cholecystitis is usually managed conservatively with rest, analgesics and antibiotics. However, suppuration of the gall bladder indicates the need for prompt surgery to either drain the gall bladder or remove it altogether. If the problem becomes a chronic disorder, surgical removal of the gall bladder (cholecystectomy) is undertaken using laparoscopic techniques. Stones within the common bile duct (choledocholithiasis) may be removed via ERCP without the need for open surgery as in former years.

PHARMACOLOGICAL FOCUS

Acute cholecystitis is a very painful condition requiring opioid analgesia and an anti-emetic. Antibiotics are also needed; one of the cephalosporins is usually prescribed, along with metronidazole if the patient is severely ill.

PRIORITIES FOR NURSING CARE

Acute Cholecystitis

- Effective pain relief (analgesia/antiemetic).
- Bed rest and assistance with personal hygiene.
- Fluid balance chart and care of IVI.
- Antibiotics and other medication as prescribed.
- Regular vital sign observations.
- Support and reassurance as the patient may be very distressed by the colicky pain.
- Early mobilization as symptoms subside.
- Education about diet and the chance to discuss long-term treatment options prior to discharge.

TEN TOP TIPS

1. Pain associated with all the conditions mentioned in this chapter is very severe so ensure that effective analgesia is given.

2. Remember to give an anti-emetic with opioid analgesia. These patients are usually feeling nauseated and vomiting is a common side effect of opioid analgesia.

3. Jaundice can have a profound effect upon a person's self concept. Offer support and talk through the symptom with the patient and family.

4. Alcohol consumption will invariably damage the liver further so use every opportunity to engage in health education about drinking.

5. Many drugs are metabolized by the liver; therapeutic doses in people with a normal liver can be toxic for a person with liver disease so be aware of side effects and ensure that a review of medications is undertaken.

6. In view of 5, educate the patient about the need to consult about over-the-counter medications (such as paracetamol) as well as prescription drugs.

7. Always follow universal precautions and full infection control procedures, especially with regard to sharps, to minimize the risk from infective hepatitis patients.

8. Jaundice causes severe itching so skin care is essential.

9. Remember the importance of fluid balance when caring for acutely ill patients.

10. Steatorrhoea is very offensive so remember the patient's embarrassment when assisting with toileting.

6

Caring for the patient with a disorder of the endocrine system

Anatomy at a glance   85
Physiology you need to know   86
Diabetes mellitus   88
Thyroid disorders   98
Other endocrine disorders   104
Ten top tips   106

ANATOMY AT A GLANCE

The endocrine system does not constitute a single organ. It consists of a series of glands scattered throughout the body whose function is to secrete hormones which are usually delivered by circulating blood to their target organs. Sometimes hormones act on neighbouring cells without needing to be carried in the blood stream, (paracrines) or even within the cell that secreted them (autocrines). Endocrine glands can either make up a whole organ as in the thyroid, or can be part of a larger organ such as the islets of Langerhans within the pancreas. Hormones regulate the functioning of their target organs and are therefore essential for the maintenance of a stable internal environment. Figure 6.1 shows some of the main endocrine glands in the body.

The endocrine system is closely linked to the nervous system and some chemical molecules can either act as a hormone or a neurotransmitter such as epinephrine (adrenaline). This neuro-endocrine linkage is closest in the hypothalamus gland, a small part of the brain inferior to the thalamus, which acts as the overall controller of the endocrine system. Adjacent to the hypothalamus is the pituitary gland, which is divided into an anterior and posterior lobe.

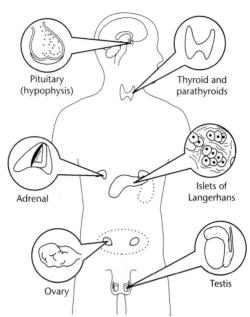

Figure 6.1 Endocrine glands in the body.

Hormones released by hypothalamus generally control the hormone secretions of the anterior lobe of pituitary gland which in turn regulate many aspects of body function.

The posterior lobe of the pituitary stores the hormones oxytocin (responsible for uterine contractions and expressing breast milk) and antidiuretic hormone (ADH or vasopressin), which acts on the renal tubules to reduce urine output and so conserve fluids, as well as having a vasoconstrictor effect.

PHYSIOLOGY YOU NEED TO KNOW (P551)

A typical example of how the hypothalamus and pituitary work together is provided by the way the hypothalamus secretes thyrotrophin-releasing hormone. This stimulates the anterior pituitary to produce thyroid-stimulating hormone (TSH), which in turn stimulates the thyroid gland to secerete the thyroid hormones T3 and T4. These hormones play a large part in controlling basal metabolic rate, and are also important in growth and development. There are six other 'releasing' hormones produced by the hypothalalmus, which stimulate the anterior pituitary to release further hormones which act elsewhere in the body. For example, the corticotropin-releasing hormone stimulates the anterior pituitary to produce the adrenocorticotropic hormone (ACTH) which in turn stimulates the adrenal glands to produce glucocorticoids such as cortisol.

Other endocrine glands function without direct control from the hypothalamus/pituitary glands, responding to changes in the internal body environment. For example, the alpha and beta cells in the islets of Langerhans (within the pancreas) secrete the hormones glucagon and insulin, respectively, to regulate blood glucose levels:

■ *Glucagon* production increases in response to a falling blood glucose level and its main effect is on liver cells leading to a breakdown of glycogen and an increase in blood glucose levels.
■ *Insulin* production increases as blood glucose levels rise. Its main effect is on muscle and adipose (fat) tissue where it promotes the removal of glucose from the blood and into the cells for storage as glycogen (muscle cells) and triglycerides (adipose tissue). In the liver, insulin promotes the utilization of glucose for energy production and storage as glycogen.

Other examples include endocrine tissue in the kidneys, which can secrete erythropoietin in response to hypoxia, resulting in increased production of red blood cells. The adrenal cortex secretes aldosterone to regulate sodium and potassium concentrations in plasma, whilst calcium levels are regulated by the release of parathormone (from the parathyroid glands) and calcitonin (from specialized cells within the thyroid).

DIABETES MELLITUS (P557)

PATHOLOGY: Key facts

Diabetes is a group of disorders of carbohydrate, fat and protein metabolism. The consequences of this disorder are profound, typically involving chronic elevated blood sugar levels (hyperglycaemia), degenerative vascular changes and damage to the nervous system (neuropathy). The damage that occurs both to the large blood vessels and the microcirculation has many serious debilitating effects. Few systems of the body escape the long-term effects of diabetes.

There are approximately 2.5 million people in the UK with diabetes and it is estimated that some 50% of people with type 2 diabetes (see below) are undiagnosed.

For this reason, diabetes is now being recognized as a major epidemic posing a serious threat to public health.

Two types of diabetes mellitus are recognized:

- *Type 1* is caused by the destruction of the beta cells in the islets of Langerhans. It is thought that this is an auto-immune response associated with genetic and environmental factors. It typically develops early in life and although the onset of symptoms can be very rapid, the destructive process may have been active for several years prior to clinical signs emerging.
- *Type 2* develops as the islets gradually reduce their output of insulin or there is increased resistance in the peripheral tissues to the action of insulin. Onset is slow and this condition is associated with obesity and lack of exercise. Although the typical age of onset is 50–70 years, the growing problem of obesity in western society is now resulting in the development of Type 2 diabetes amongst children and young adults who are seriously overweight. There is also a strong genetic influence with Type 2 diabetes being far more common in some families and in certain ethnic groups. For example, in the UK, Pakistanis and Bangladeshis are five times more likely than the general population to develop Type 2 diabetes, whilst Indians are three times more likely.

Effects on the Patient

■ Immediate:

- Hyperglycaemia.
- Increased fat metabolism as a substitute source of energy may lead to increasing levels of ketone bodies in the blood (ketoacidosis).
- Proteins may also be broken down to amino acids for gluconeogenesis leading to further rises in blood sugar levels and body wasting.
- Increased output of urine (polyuria) due to the increased concentration of glucose in the glomerular filtrate in the kidneys. This leads to dehydration and electrolyte imbalance. Glucose is found in the urine (glucosuria).

■ Long-term effects are many and varied. The following list notes only the more common:

- Microvascular degenerative changes affecting the skin, kidneys and retinas.
- Retinopathy or minute aneurysms in the retinal blood vessels which are prone to rupture. This ultimately leads to blindness.
- Cataract formation.
- Renal failure caused by changes in the glomerular capillaries and larger blood vessels.
- Macrovascular degenerative changes associated with the deposition of cholesterol in the arteries, narrowing their lumen and reducing blood supply to the distal organ. This can lead to angina or myocardial infarction if the coronary arteries are involved or if the vessels supplying blood to the legs are affected, this leads to peripheral vascular disease, gangrene and potentially amputation of the limb.
- Diabetic neuropathy affecting the peripheral nervous system and typically leading to abnormal burning feelings or loss of sensation in the lower limbs.

■ Acute metabolic emergencies:

- *Diabetic ketoacidosis.* This life-threatening complication develops insidiously over a few days and is associated with inadequate insulin levels and rising blood glucose concentrations. Ketones accumulate in the blood making the patient acidotic, dehydration develops because of the kidney's increased urine output caused by the elevated glucose levels; the patient also loses sodium and potassium. The severity of this condition is not related to the blood glucose levels, and the patient may be awake and conscious although feeling unwell. The classic 'diabetic coma' is a rare event. The pulse tends to be rapid with a low blood pressure. In severe cases, where the patient's level of consciousness is seriously affected, breathing is often of a deep sighing nature as the person attempts to correct for the acidosis by excreting as much carbon dioxide as possible.

● *Hyperglycaemic hyperosmolar non-ketotic diabetic coma.* This situation develops if blood glucose levels climb but the person's metabolism does not produce excess ketone bodies. The person is therefore not severely acidotic. It often happens in older people with Type 2 diabetes and blood glucose levels can be extremely high with profound dehydration and hypovolaemia (shock) eventually leading to confusion and coma as fluid shifts from the intracellular into the extracellular spaces. This condition has a high mortality rate.

● *Hypoglycaemia.* In this situation, the patient's blood glucose levels fall dangerously low usually owing to inappropriate self medication and nutrition or excess exercise. Early signs are of confusion, drowsiness, unsteadiness. The person may appear drunk – an easy mistake to make for a lay person who does not know the patient.

WHAT TO LOOK OUT FOR

Type 1 and Type 2 diabetes tend to have different presentations and these are summarized in Table 6.1.

The diagnosis of diabetes is made from:

■ The classic symptoms of Type 1 diabetes such as thirst, polyuria and unexplained weight loss.

■ A casual plasma glucose level >11.1 mmol/L ('casual' means taken at any time).

■ Or a fasting blood glucose >7.0 mmol/L ('fasting' means no food in previous 8 hours).

Table 6.1 Classification of diabetes mellitus

	Type 1	Type 2
Synonyms	Juvenile onset	Maturity onset
Age of onset	Usually before 30 years	Usually after 40 years
Type of onset	Frequently sudden	Usually gradual
Presentation	Polydipsia, polyuria	Often asymptomatic
Bodyweight	Thin	Usually (80%) obese
Ketoacidosis	Ketosis-prone	Ketosis-resistant
Control of diabetes	Difficulty; brittle	Generally easy
Control by diet alone	Not possible	Frequently possible
Control by oral agents	Not possible	Frequently possible
Long-term complications	Frequent	Frequent

- Many patients with Type 2 diabetes do not present with the classic signs of Type 1, and the diagnosis may be made from a random urine test or capillary blood test carried out as part of a general health assessment.
- Type 2 diabetes may present in a middle-aged patient who is complaining of generally feeling unwell and tired all the time but with no specific symptoms.
- Type 2 diabetes may be discovered in the patient whose presentation is due to symptoms of long-term complications such as angina, eye problems or peripheral vascular disease.
- Pruritus of the vulva due to infection associated with glucose deposited from the urine. Males may complain of a swollen and inflamed glans penis (balanitis) due to the same effect.
- Microalbuminuria or proteinuria may be detected upon dipstix testing of the urine. These are serious indicators of developing vascular complications of diabetes.

■ Diabetic ketoacidosis:
  ● Anorexia, nausea and vomiting.
  ● Drowsiness, fatigue.
  ● Signs of dehydration.
■ As the disorder develops:
  ● Increasing depth and rate of respirations.
  ● Rapid thready pulse, falling blood pressure (BP).
  ● Abdominal pains.
  ● Finally coma. Note that coma is the end stage of a process that may take several days to develop, although it can occur with greater rapidity.
■ Hypoglycaemia:
  ● Sweating and tremors.
  ● Weakness, tachycardia.
  ● Signs of apprehension and anxiety.
  ● Later signs include confusion, unsteady gait, clumsiness and dizziness as the brain becomes increasingly affected by falling blood sugar levels.
  ● Convulsions and coma are late signs of a fully developed crisis.

MEDICAL MANAGEMENT

The aims of management are to establish and maintain good metabolic control. This will avoid life-threatening crises such as ketoacidosis, allow the person to live as normal a life as possible, and prolong life by preventing long-term complications. Many of the interventions aimed at producing these desirable outcomes fall within the nursing sphere of responsibility (e.g. lifestyle modification, weight reduction, smoking cessation, diet and exercise), and will be discussed shortly.

Drug therapy and dietary control are the mainstays of management, aiming to keep blood glucose within normal limits. Many patients can be managed without insulin, utilizing drugs known as oral hypoglycaemics (see the next section).

It is now thought that the tighter the control of blood glucose levels, the lower the risk from long-term complications. Medical management therefore assesses diabetic control by measuring concentrations of a fraction of the haemoglobin molecule known as glycated haemoglobin (HbA$_{1c}$). Measurements of this fraction of haemoglobin give a reliable estimate of average blood glucose levels over the preceding 6–8 weeks. This can be used to check against the self-assessed capillary blood glucose results that the patient has been recording in their diary. It is possible that patients who are not adhering to their medication and dietary regimens may falsify results leading all concerned to an inaccurate view of the extent of metabolic control. This deception can be very damaging to the patient in the long term, and needs to be (tactfully) challenged if detected. It is, however, a delicate balancing act between tight glycaemic control and avoiding the risk of hypoglycaemic episodes.

If the patient presents in a ketoacidotic condition, this is a medical emergency, and the priorities are to rehydrate the patient rapidly with IV fluids and restore electrolyte balance, especially potassium, which may be dangerously depleted. Insulin will also be given intravenously to restore blood glucose levels to normal.

Serum lipids, total cholesterol, low density lipoprotein cholesterol and triglyceride are measured regularly as this information provides important information about overall metabolic control. This information is particularly important given the linkage with cardiovascular complications.

Regular monitoring of the patient's urine for signs of proteinuria (dipstix) or microalbuminuria (involving 24-hour urine collections) are carried out to detect early signs of renal involvement.

In recent years, there has been a trend away from hospital outpatient clinics for the management of stable diabetic patients. Increasingly, this role has been carried out in primary care by GPs working with specialist nurses or nurse practitioners who can refer to a hospital consultant should the need arise.

PHARMACOLOGY FOCUS

Insulin

This medication is required by those who cannot maintain normal blood glucose levels by a combination of diet and oral hypoglycaemic medication. It is also given in emergencies such as diabetic ketoacidosis. Most insulin used today is prepared synthetically by genetic engineering and various preparations are available which differ in their speed and duration of action. In addition, biphasic insulins are used which are a mixture of a rapid acting insulin and one of long duration (e.g. Humalog Mix 25 or Human Mixtard). This gives the obvious benefit of a quick action which is then prolonged in effect.

Insulin dosage is measured in units and each individual's regime is prepared in conjunction with their diet and daily activity. The aim is to maximize insulin activity after major meals and to provide a steady overnight action. It may take some time and experimentation for a newly diagnosed diabetic to arrive at a diet and insulin regime that gives the best results for that person.

Insulin is a protein and therefore would be digested and destroyed if given orally. It is therefore given by subcutaneous injection, the preferred sites are shown in Figure 6.2. The skin needs to be clean but there is no need to swab with an alcohol wipe. The injection should be at 90 degrees to the skin, using disposable insulin syringes which have the needle attached already to the syringe. One site at a time should be used with each injection approximately 2.5 cm from the previous one until the whole site is used and then another site should be used. This rotation prevents the development of scarring and fibrosis. Apart from being unsightly, damaged areas do not absorb insulin rapidly and smoothly, reducing the effectiveness of the injection.

Oral Hypoglycaemic Agents

Type 2 diabetes can be controlled in most people by diet and several other types of drugs other than insulin, all of which can be given orally, hence this collective name.

- *Sulphonylureas* stimulate beta cells in the islets of Langerhans to produce more insulin, e.g. glibenclamide, gliclazide.
- *Biguanides* reduce the production of glucose in the liver and increase its uptake in muscle. The patient has to be manufacturing some insulin for this drug to work. Metformin is the only member of this group licensed in the

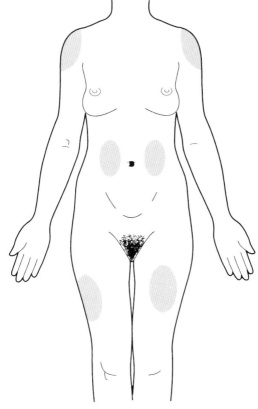

Figure 6.2 Sites for insulin injection.

UK and it may be combined with a non-sulfonylurea insulin secretagogue (nateglinide) which increases insulin secretion in the presence of food.

■ *Meglitinides* such as repaglinide taken just before a meal can enhance the effect of metformin.

■ *Thiazolidinediones* increase the sensitivity of cells to insulin and so can be used in conjunction with either a sulphonylurea or metformin (e.g. rosiglitazone or pioglitazone).

PRIORITIES FOR NURSING CARE

Patient education is a major nursing role, covering many areas besides those listed below.

■ *Diet.* Patients are encouraged to work with the dietician and other clinical staff to develop their own diet that ensures good blood glucose level control. A plan indicates the expected number of calories per day and how these should be distributed between fats (30%), carbohydrates (55–60%) and proteins (12–20%). If the patient is overweight, the dietary plan requires weight loss therefore total calories should be less than required for normal everyday activity. Particular attention is paid to:

● Unrefined carbohydrates high in fibre are especially beneficial e.g. wholegrain bread, cereals, fruit and vegetables and these should replace refined carbohydrates.

● Foods high in soluble fibre such as oats, rice, legumes and lentils reduce glycaemia and low-density lipoprotein (LDL) levels.

● Ensuring that carbohydrate intake is distributed throughout the day to avoid sharp peaks in glucose concentrations.

● Unsaturated fats substituted for saturated fats because of the high risk of atherosclerosis and vascular lesions in diabetes.

Key dietary factors are summarized in Box 6.1.

■ *Medication.* A great deal of teaching is required to ensure that the patient who is dependent upon insulin understands how it works, their dosage and injection technique. Similarly, the patient on oral hypoglycaemics needs to understand their medication, and both groups of patients need to be aware of the signs of an accidental hypoglycaemic attack. Their relatives and carers also need to be aware of this problem and the measures that will correct a 'hypo'.

■ *Accurate monitoring* of blood glucose levels by use of the correct technique and maintenance of a diary of readings. Urine glucose measurements are not very reliable as different people have different threshold values above which glucose appears in the blood. Additionally, urine monitoring gives no indication of low blood sugar levels.

Box 6.1 Key points regarding diet for the person with diabetes mellitus

- ■ The diet provides approximately 45–60% of calories as carbohydrate, no more than 1 g/kg body weight protein and less than 35% as fat (emphasis on monounsaturated fat)
- ■ Total calorie intake will be adjusted as necessary for the individual to achieve and maintain a desirable weight
- ■ Calorie intake is adequate to provide for optimal growth and development (childhood, pregnancy and lactation)
- ■ Carbohydrate intake is evenly distributed throughout the day and consistent from day to day.
- ■ The diet should consist of normal foods, with a preference for foods that contain unrefined carbohydrates and are high in soluble fibre
- ■ Food intake is adjusted to accommodate changes in lifestyle (e.g. illness, physical activity, emotional stress, eating out and travel)
- ■ Meal plans are individualized and consider social, cultural and ethnic values of the patient and family

- ■ *Management of hypoglycaemia.* In most cases, simple measures such as a rapid intake of two or three sugar cubes, a sweet drink (tea or coffee) with 2–3 spoons of sugar or 2–3 spoonfuls of honey will suffice. If this does not produce an improvement, one unit of glucagon should be given immediately, injected via the intramuscular or subcutaneous route and a 999 call made. Paramedics can administer IV glucose if the patient has not improved when they arrive.
- ■ *Avoidance of hypoglycaemia* by regular monitoring of capillary blood glucose levels and regulation of diet, exercise and insulin intake including reducing insulin dosage before extended exercise such as sport.
- ■ *Skin care.* The diabetic person's risk of neuropathy and circulatory problems make careful skin care essential, particularly of the feet. Any small lesion can quickly become infected leading to septicaemia and/or gangrene.
- ■ *Regular eye checks*, at least once a year, are essential due to the potential for serious ophthalmic problems.

■ *Lifestyle modification.* Patient teaching and coaching are essential to try and secure smoking cessation, increased levels of exercise and weight reduction, particularly with Type 2 diabetics. Young adults diagnosed with Type 1 diabetes present a different set of challenges as peer group pressure is often difficult to reconcile with the restrictions upon lifestyle that are necessary, leading to poor metabolic control.

■ *Pregnancy* is a hazardous undertaking for a diabetic woman and careful consideration is needed before embarking upon a family.

THYROID DISORDERS (P576)

PATHOLOGY: Key facts

Disorder of the thyroid can lead to undersecretion (hypothyroidism) or oversecretion of the thyroid hormones (hyperthyroidism) with far-reaching effects upon the person. A key element in the production of the thyroid hormones (T3 and T4) is iodine, which is concentrated and stored in the thyroid gland. Lack of iodine in the diet can therefore cause hypothyroidism. Environmental escapes of radioactive iodine isotopes from nuclear accidents can cause serious damage to the thyroid such as cancer although paradoxically, in controlled low doses, a radioactive isotope of iodine (^{131}I) is very effective in treating hyperthyroidism.

Hypothyroidism

■ Commonly affects older people, women are approximately six times as likely as men to be affected.

■ Most common causes are an autoimmune disorder (Hashimoto's disease) or excess destruction of thyroid tissue in treatment of hyperthyroidism.

■ A child may be born with congenital hypothyroidism resulting in failure to thrive, stunted growth and profound learning disability unless recognized and treated promptly with thyroid hormones.

■ A less common cause is iodine deficiency resulting in an enlarged thyroid known as a goitre.

Hyperthyroidism

- Graves disease is the most common form of this disorder involving well-defined ophthalmic pathology (exophthalmus). It is an autoimmune disorder affecting the whole thyroid and affects women far more than men. Localized adenomas may over-produce thyroxin giving rise to 'toxic goitre' but the ophthalmic pathology associated with Graves disease is absent.
- Hyperthyroidism affects females more than males and is commonest in the age range 30–60, although toxic adenoma is more common in older people.

WHAT TO LOOK OUT FOR

The clinical characteristics of the two main thyroid disorders are caused by either excess or insufficient production of the thyroid hormones. This leads to disturbance of basal metabolism, activity, mental functioning, sex drive and dysfunction of the integumentary system (skin, hair, etc.), which are all subject to thyroid hormone control. These changes are summarized in Table 6.2.

MEDICAL MANAGEMENT

Hypothyroidism

Treatment consists of thyroxine tablets to replace the thyroid hormones which the person is unable to produce. Therapy starts on low doses which are gradually built up over the first few weeks. Patients generally report feeling better within 2–3 weeks but it may be several months before skin and hair texture return to normal. Obesity is common and weight loss may prove very difficult even with long-term hormone replacement therapy.

Hyperthyroidism

There are three main approaches:

- Antithyroid drugs (e.g. carbimazole) which suppress thyroid function are usually given to younger patients experiencing their first episode.
- Surgery (subtotal thyroidectomy) for those experiencing recurrence despite antithyroid drug therapy or for more severe cases, especially in males.

Table 6.2 Assessment of the person with altered thyroid function

	Clinical characteristics	
	Hypothyroidism	Hyperthyroidism
Nutrition and metabolism	Pulse rate decreased	Pulse rapid and bounding
	Blood pressure low	Palpitations
	Respirations decreased	Increased blood pressure
	Appetite poor	Respiratory rate increased
	Weight gain	Appetite increased
	Serum cholesterol raised	Weight loss
		Serum cholesterol decreased
Activity tolerance	Weakness and fatigue	Weakness and fatigue
	Slow movements	Weakness of eyelid muscles
	Dyspnoea	Shortness of breath on exertion
	Decreased muscle tone and reflexes	Tremor of hands
	Increased muscle tone and reflexes	
Skin integrity	Skin dry, thick and pale	Increased sweating
	Eyelids oedematous	Skin warm and moist
	Lips and tongue enlarged	Eyelids retracted
	Hair coarse and sparse	Hair loss
	Interstitial oedema	

Thought processes and emotional responses	Slow mental processes	Anxiety, apprehension
	Increased sleep and lethargy	Restlessness
	Speech hoarse, slow and monotonous	Irritability
	Depression	Emotional instability
	Mental disturbance	Insomnia
Bowel elimination	Decreased gastrointestinal motility	Increased gastrointestinal motility
	Constipation	Diarrhoea
Thermoregulation	Sensitivity to cold	Sensitivity to heat
	Decreased body temperature	Increased body temperature
Sexuality patterns	Metrorrhagia	Oligomenorrhoea or amenorrhoea
	Amenorrhoea	Low sex drive
	Low sex drive	Impotence
	Infertility	

■ Radioactive iodine (isotope ^{131}I) is given orally and becomes concentrated in the thyroid gland where it destroys thyroid cells and inhibits their ability to replicate. This approach tends to be used for older patients and for those in which other approaches have failed.

PHARMACOLOGY FOCUS

The antithyroid drugs such as carbimazole can produce agranulocytosis as a side effect, therefore the patient should be warned to seek medical help should they develop a sore throat, swollen neck glands, fever or any rash. Beta blockers may also be given in the short term to reduce the stimulating effect on the heart of excess thyroxin production.

PRIORITIES FOR NURSING CARE

Hypothyroidism

■ Considerable psychological support to both patient and family is needed as the patient may be withdrawn, apathetic and suffer from self neglect due to the effects of this condition. The patient may initially be very slow and dull, requiring a great deal of patience, until the thyroid hormone replacement therapy begins to work.

■ Extra clothing and heating are needed.

■ Skin care should involve using the minimum of soap but dryness should be relieved with oils and creams.

■ Obesity commonly develops so a low-calorie diet is important to begin weight loss.

■ Fluids should be encouraged with high-fibre diet to prevent constipation.

■ Patient/family teaching about the disorder and the long-term medication (thyroid hormone replacement therapy) required.

Hyperthyroidism

■ Education about the disorder and the treatment regime that is to be undertaken are essential to gain the understanding and cooperation of patient and family.

■ Anxiety and stress should be reduced by talking through the disorder and providing a quiet stress-free environment, whether at home or on the ward. Activity needs to be reduced by trying to engage the patient in activities that expend little energy.

■ Weight loss needs to be corrected and the person restored to a normal weight for their height/gender through a high-protein, high-carbohydrate, high-calorie diet.

■ Fluid intake should be increased because of the high metabolic rate (3000 mL/day).

■ Skin and eye care are essential to prevent complications.

The patient undergoing surgery will need the standard care for any patient undergoing a general anaesthetic and surgery. In addition they will need:

■ A careful explanation about the procedure, including reassurance that the incision will be made in such a way as to have the minimum visual impact upon the neck.

■ Careful positioning and support for the neck post-operatively together with monitoring of breathing because of the risk of airway obstruction from tissue swelling.

■ Drainage from neck drains should be monitored carefully to avoid the risk of a haematoma forming which could obstruct the airway.

■ Gradual mobilization of the head and neck region. The area will be painful and stiff while the patient may be very apprehensive about moving their neck for fear of damaging the wound. Exercises prescribed by the physiotherapist should be encouraged.

■ Encouragement with a soft diet before progressing on to solids as swallowing may be painful at first.

■ Monitoring for complications of surgery which although rare can be very serious:

 ● Bleeding around the neck region may lead to shock and occlusion of the airway.

 ● Injury to one of the recurrent laryngeal nerves during surgery may lead to hoarseness and a weak voice but if both are damaged this can lead to paralysis of the muscles on both sides of the larynx and respiratory obstruction.

 ● Parathyroid damage may lead to a reduction in parathormone levels and hence serum calcium levels which in turn causes tetany, a state of heightened neuromuscular irritability. The patient complains of pins and needles or tingling sensations together with muscle spasm and cramp-like pains.

- An acute episode of thyrotoxicosis rarely may occur as a result of a sudden release of thyroid hormones caused by the surgical intervention.

■ Frequent vital signs observations with particular attention being paid to the airway and respiration are therefore crucial in the period immediately after surgery.

The person undergoing radio-iodine treatment will need reassurance as many people may be alarmed at the prospect of taking a medication that is radioactive. The patient is not a radiation hazard to other people or nursing staff as the radiation levels are so low. However, this treatment is never given if the patient is pregnant. The patient should be monitored for signs of inflammation of the gland such as soreness and redness and any signs of subsequent thyroid disorder. The practice nurse or outpatients nurses are usually involved in this follow-up care.

OTHER ENDOCRINE DISORDERS (P585)

Diabetes and thyroid disorders account for the vast majority of endocrine diseases encountered in primary care or on a general hospital medical ward. Fortunately, other conditions are rare and often treated at specialist centres. The principal disorders are listed below:

Parathyroid Gland

■ Hyperparathyroidism leads to decalcification and weakening of bone, muscle weakness, increased serum calcium levels and increased risk of renal calculi.

■ Hypothyroidism leads to low serum calcium levels, muscle spasm and tetany.

Pituitary Gland

■ Oversecretion of growth hormone before the fusion of the epiphyses produces gigantism whilst after skeletal maturity it produces acromegaly (thickening of bones, growth of cartilage, enlargement of the head, hands and feet).

■ Simmond's disease occurs when there is a complete failure of the anterior pituitary to produce any hormones resulting in lack of stimulation to the thyroid, adrenal cortices and gonads leading to wasting, the appearance of rapid ageing, hypoglycaemia, hypotension and coma.

■ Diabetes insipidus occurs when part of the hypothalamic – pituitary system is destroyed by neoplasm, infection or brain injury. As a result there is a deficiency of anti-diuretic hormone (ADH) leading to profound dehydration and electrolyte imbalance caused by a urinary output of between 5 and 20 L/day.

■ The syndrome of inappropriate production of antidiuretic hormone refers to overproduction of ADH. The result is water intoxication increasing blood volume and haemodilution but sodium depletion. Decreasing level of consciousness and seizures develop as a result of effects of water intoxication on the brain.

Adrenal Gland

■ Adrenal insufficiency results from inadequate secretion of cortisol and/or aldosterone and is potentially fatal. The most common cause is inappropriate withdrawal of long-term glucocorticoid therapy or a pituitary tumour leading to ACTH deficiency and a lack of glucocorticoids. Adrenal cortex disorder can produce Addison's disease (inadequate production of corticosteroids), a rare but potentially fatal disease.

■ Cushing's syndrome (excess corticosteroid production) is usually caused by long-term steroid therapy. It may arise as a primary disorder due to excess ACTH production from a pituitary tumour leading to bilateral adrenal hyperplasia. Women are four times more likely than men to develop this condition which has a 50% 5-year mortality.

■ A neoplasm of the adrenal medulla is known as a phaeochromocytoma and results in excess production of epinephrine and norepinephrine leading to very high blood pressure, hyperglycaemia and general hypermetabolism.

TEN TOP TIPS

1. Diabetes is a complex metabolic disorder that affects the *whole* body; remember this whenever talking to a diabetic patient about health education.
2. 50% of people with Type 2 diabetes are unaware they have the disorder so consider Type 2 diabetes when assessing middle-aged patients, especially if overweight or complaining of feeling unwell/tired all the time.
3. Capillary blood glucose testing is one of the foundations of diabetes management; make sure you are using the equipment properly and in line with manufacturer's instructions.
4. Try and encourage diabetic patients to give up smoking; it is never too late.
5. Be aware of the early signs of hypoglycaemia.
6. Ensure that insulin is stored at the correct temperature and is not past its 'use by' date.
7. Make sure you can give patients a sensible account of their oral hypoglycaemic medication and side effects to watch out for.
8. Be able to give a concise account of what constitutes a good diet and exercise regime for a diabetic patient. You may have to do this in response to a question from a patient or family member without any prior notice so sound authoritative and get it right!
9. Hypothyroid patients can present in primary care with a range of symptoms from depression, tired all the time to being worried about their weight.
10. Know the complications of thyroid surgery; although very rare, they can have disastrous consequences if not spotted promptly.

Caring for the patient with a disorder of the urinary system

Anatomy at a glance 107
Physiology you need to know 109
Urinary tract infection 111
Incontinence 113
Benign prostatic hyperplasia 116
Prostate cancer 118
Chronic kidney disease and renal failure 120
Acute renal failure 120
Chronic kidney disease/renal failure 122
Ten top tips 125

ANATOMY AT A GLANCE

The kidneys are retroperitoneal (i.e. posterior to the peritoneum) and extend from the 12th thoracic to the third lumbar vertebra. They are approximately 10–12 cm long, 5–7 cm wide and 3 cm thick, and are partly protected by the 11th and 12th pairs of ribs.

Each kidney consists of a fatty capsule containing the medulla and cortex, which collectively is known as the renal parenchyma (see Figure 7.1). The medulla is divided up into a series of subunits known as the renal pyramids (between 8 and 18 per kidney). The functional units of the kidneys are the nephrons, which are contained within the medulla and cortex, totalling approximately one million per kidney.

- *Blood supply*: as can be seen from Figure 7.2, each nephron is supplied with blood via an afferent arteriole, which divides into a tangled web of capillaries called the glomerulus before reuniting to form an efferent arteriole

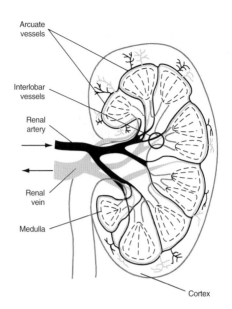

Figure 7.1 Cross-section of the kidney.

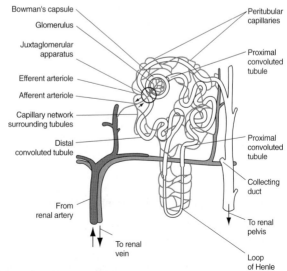

Figure 7.2 A renal unit, or nephron, of the cortex of the kidney.

that is narrower than the original afferent arteriole. The efferent arteriole then subdivides into a network of peritubular capillaries, which surrounds the tubule before reuniting to form the peritubular venules which feed into the renal vein.

■ *The nephron*: the glomerulus is surrounded by a capsule which leads into the tubule itself. The tubule has four portions:
  ● Proximal convoluted tubule
  ● Loop of Henle
  ● Distal convoluted tubule
  ● Collecting duct.

■ *The ureters*: the urine drains via the collecting ducts eventually into the minor calyces and finally into the calyx of the kidney and on into the ureter at the pelvis of the kidney. The ureter is a 25–30 cm long tube consisting of involuntary muscle which carries the urine to the bladder. Gravity and waves of peristalsis spreading through the muscle wall of the ureter propel urine to the bladder.

■ *The bladder*: this consists of a muscular sac with a capacity of 700–800 mL which stores urine ready for excretion. The muscle in the bladder wall is arranged in three layers, and is collectively known as the detrusor muscle. The ureters enter through the bladder wall at an oblique angle, relying on the pressure of urine in a filling bladder to compress the ureters and so close them sufficiently to prevent backflow into the kidney (there is no valve system to prevent backflow).

■ *The urethra*: the internal sphincter of the bladder (involuntary muscle) and external sphincter (voluntary muscle) guard the entrance to the urethra. In females the urethra is very short (4 cm), but may be 15–20 cm in males. The urethra empties via the external urinary meatus.

PHYSIOLOGY YOU NEED TO KNOW

As adults we are 55% (women) to 60% (men) water. Some 66% of that water resides within cells and is known as intracellular fluid; the rest is extracellular fluid divided between plasma and interstitial fluid in a ratio of about 1:4. We excrete an average of 1500 mL of urine per day, but also lose some 600 mL of water in evaporation from the skin, 300 mL in breathing out and a further 100 mL in faecal matter. Fluid intake therefore needs to be around 2500 mL per day to achieve fluid balance.

The functions of the renal system may be summarized as follows:

■ To regulate fluid and electrolyte balance within the body. This ensures that
  ● Electrolyte concentrations stay within their normal ranges (e.g. sodium, potassium, chloride, calcium, phosphates).
  ● Blood volume is kept within normal limits.
  ● Blood osmolarity is maintained (a measure of the total number of dissolved particles per litre of solution) ensuring that osmosis helps maintain the balance between the different fluid compartments of the body.
  ● Blood pressure is maintained within normal limits.
  ● The acid–base balance (pH) is maintained.
■ To produce renin, which helps maintain blood pressure via the angiotensin pathway.
■ Removal of the waste products of metabolism such as urea, ammonia, etc.
■ Production of erythropoietin which stimulates red bone marrow to produce red blood cells.
■ Assists in the production of vitamin D (calcitrol) which helps the body extract calcium from food in the gut.

The kidneys achieve this complex range of functions by filtering the blood as it passes through each nephron, selectively reabsorbing substances the body needs to conserve, including large amounts of water and secreting the waste products of metabolism into the tubular filtrate as it passes to the collecting ducts.

■ *Filtration*: occurs in the glomerulus, the narrower diameter efferent arteriole helps generate filtration pressure within the glomerulus as does overall blood pressure. Filtration rate depends largely on the rate of supply of blood to the kidneys via the renal arteries. Average rate is 105–125 mL/min.

- *Reabsorption*: this occurs as molecules move from the filtrate through the wall of the tubule into the interstitial fluid, and finally into the network of tubular blood vessels. The proximal convoluted tubule sees the reabsorption of large quantities of glucose, sodium, potassium, chloride and water, to name but a few substances. Lesser amounts of water, sodium, potassium and chloride are absorbed in the loop of Henle and further small amounts of water, sodium and chloride in the distal convoluted tubule.

- *Secretion*: waste products such as urea, creatinine, ammonium and free hydrogen ions are secreted into the filtrate on its passage through the tubule. The body may fine-tune water and potassium reabsorption in the final part of the distal tubule and collecting duct. The hormone aldosterone acts here to secrete excess potassium into the filtrate for excretion and reabsorb sodium and water in return. Antidiuretic hormone can increase the rate of water reabsorption in this final region of the nephron, concentrating the urine further.

- *Micturition*: occurs when the bladder walls become stretched as the bladder fills with 200–400 mL of urine. Nerve impulses are conducted to the micturition centre of the spinal cord (S2 and S3 segments), where a reflex arc produces reflex contraction of the detrusor muscle in the wall of the bladder. However, as adults we are able to override this reflex emptying urge through our conscious control of the voluntary, external urinary sphincter muscle. This is a skill that young children have to learn around the age of 2–3 years to achieve continence.

URINARY TRACT INFECTION (P641)

PATHOLOGY: Key facts

Infection and inflammation of the urethra is called urethritis, and when the bladder is involved, cystitis. Approximately, 20% of women will experience at least one episode of urinary tract infection (UTI). This high incidence is thought to be due to the short female urethra (4 cm) making the entry of organisms from the rectum (e.g. *Escherichia coli*) and vagina much easier. Poor toilet hygiene and sexual activity increase the risk of infection, as does the presence of an indwelling urinary catheter or compression of the bladder by the uterus during pregnancy. UTI is much rarer in men, although men aged over 65 developing urinary obstructive problems due to an enlarged prostate are prone to UTI.

WHAT TO LOOK OUT FOR

The person complains of frequency and dysuria (soreness or discomfort on passing urine). Urine may be foul smelling, look cloudy (due to cell casts and pus) and test positive with a dipstix to protein and/or blood. It may also have an alkaline pH.

MEDICAL MANAGEMENT

Culture and sensitivity of urine will determine the organism causing the UTI. If the condition does not respond to antimicrobial treatment immediately, this implies that the UTI may be secondary to some other problem, and further investigations are carried out. Bladder calculi, urethral stricture or pyelonephritis (infection of the kidney itself) are possibilities, while in men, obstructive prostatic problems need to be checked for.

PHARMACOLOGY FOCUS

In the majority of cases, an uncomplicated UTI will be treated with a 3-day course of trimethoprim. If this does not clear the UTI, the culture and sensitivity results will guide prescription of second-line antimicrobial drugs. Drug resistance is becoming more of a problem as strains of organisms such as *E. coli* develop resistance to the common antimicrobial drugs.

PRIORITIES FOR NURSING CARE

The focus is on preventing UTI:

■ Scrupulous hand washing and cross-infection prevention measures.

- Patient education about personal hygiene associated with defecation (wipe from front to rear and wash hands thoroughly) and sex (*both* partners should wash their hands and genitals thoroughly before sex and, if problems persist, use condoms).
- Drinking large amounts of fluid helps dilute urine and prevent a build-up in concentration of organisms; citrus fruit juices may also assist.

If the patient has an indwelling catheter:

- A closed drainage system is essential.
- Urine specimens should only be obtained using a sterile needle via sampling port.
- Wash hands and wear gloves when handling any of the equipment.
- Do not allow the drainage bag tap to come in contact with any other objects.

There is no evidence to support the use of:

1. Antiseptic creams/lotions applied to the external urinary meatus to reduce the risk of UTI.
2. The addition of bactericidal agents to urine drainage bags to reduce UTI risk.
3. Bladder installations to maintain catheter patency by dissolving encrustations.

INCONTINENCE (P633)

PATHOLOGY: Key facts

Urinary incontinence is still a difficult and embarrassing subject for many people to talk about, despite the fact that it affects millions of people in the UK. Various estimates give figures in the region of 25–30% of women being affected at some stage in their lives, while older men in particular also experience problems.

Physiological Causes

- Instability of the bladder wall muscle (the detrusor muscle) causes spontaneous bladder contraction and emptying with little or no warning.

■ Stress incontinence occurs mostly in females after child-bearing leading to laxity of pelvic floor muscles. Any sudden increase in bladder pressure (such as caused by sneezing or laughing) leads to expulsion of urine.

■ Spinal cord damage interfering with nerve control of bladder function.

■ Retention with overflow. In this situation the bladder fills up with urine which cannot be excreted normally (e.g. due to prostatic obstruction). Pressure within the bladder eventually forces the urinary sphincters open and some urine escapes (incontinence) but as pressure falls no further urine can escape and a large residual volume is left in the bladder (retention).

Extrinsic Causes

■ Limited mobility and dexterity may mean that although a patient is aware of the need to micturate, they cannot make it to the toilet in time.

■ Confusion.

■ Low expectations of carers leads to avoidable episodes of incontinence.

Intrinsic Causes

■ Faecal impaction compressing the bladder.

■ UTI or the polyuria of diabetes can contribute to incontinence problems.

WHAT TO LOOK OUT FOR

Patients are very embarrassed about urinary incontinence, and may be reluctant to admit to such a problem. You need to be aware of tell-tale signs, such as the smell of stale urine or stains on furniture in a person's own home. It may be more subtle than that, however, and the only clue may be withdrawal from social activity as an elderly person fears the embarrassment of incontinence.

MEDICAL MANAGEMENT

Many people with incontinence can be helped and their quality of life greatly improved by positive medical and nursing intervention. Investigations to determine the cause of the problem come first. These include a midstream specimen of urine for culture and sensitivity, residual volume determination, urodynamic investigations measuring urine flows and pressures, and keeping a diary of voiding and continence.

Medical intervention occurs when there is an obvious cause amenable to medical intervention such as benign prostatic hypertrophy (surgery) or a urinary tract infection (antimicrobial therapy). Expert nursing care combined with physiotherapy/occupational therapy is often the main line of management once the cause of the problem has been determined (see below).

PHARMACOLOGY FOCUS

Anticholinergic drugs (e.g. tolterodine) may be used to treat detrusor muscle instability in the bladder wall (urge incontinence).

PRIORITIES FOR NURSING CARE

- Pelvic floor exercises can greatly improve stress incontinence problems.
- A bladder training programme starts by keeping an accurate voiding diary for several days. This establishes the pattern for the individual and allows a schedule for toilet visits to be devised, initially every 1–2 hours. Physical activity is encouraged and fluid intake of at least 2000 mL/day is required to avoid dehydration and increased risk of UTI.
- If patients have very short notice of voiding (urge incontinence) always ensure that appliances are readily available or that they are sitting within easy access of a toilet. Modifications of clothing to replace difficult buttons and zippers with velcro may also help maintain continence.
- Various protective pads and appliances are available where continence cannot be regained. Catheterization may be used as a means of controlling incontinence. Complications such as catheters blocking with encrustations, falling out or giving rise to UTI mean catheterization should not be considered until other methods have been tried. The catheter can either be left indwelling or introduced intermittently to drain the bladder. External urinary drainage

devices (condom and collecting bag) are very useful for men as they are non-invasive. The penis must be regularly inspected for redness and excoriation.

Close collaboration with the departments of physiotherapy and occupational therapy is necessary to help many patients. Review of medication with medical staff is also beneficial as older patients in particular may be on many different medications which can be exacerbating the problem (such as diuretics).

BENIGN PROSTATIC HYPERPLASIA (P774)

PATHOLOGY: Key facts

Enlargement of the prostate gland occurs in most men as part of the ageing process and is caused by an imbalance in androgen/oestrogen, levels. Approximately 50% of men over 50 will have some degree of benign prostatic hyperplasia (BPH) and 10–30% of men in their early 70s are symptomatic. As the gland enlarges it causes obstruction to the outflow of urine from the bladder. Eventually this may cause the retention of a large volume of residual urine which is prone to become infected, retention with overflow problems and possibly acute and complete retention of urine. This last condition leads to a distended abdomen and severe pain. Acute retention is often provoked by alcohol or drugs such as antidepressants, tranquillizers or antimuscarinic drugs such as ipratropium.

WHAT TO LOOK OUT FOR

The onset of the condition is insidious. The man may notice increasing difficulty starting to void, a poor stream, dribbling and frequency, especially at night where sleep is disturbed. Signs of a UTI may be present if there is significant residual urine. Acute retention of urine is very distressing and painful as the man may give a history of drinking normally but not being able to pass urine for 12 hours or more. An obvious distension of the lower abdomen is usually present. In carrying out a health assessment of any man over 50 years of age, the nurse should always check for symptoms of BPH as it is such a widespread disorder and one that many men feel embarrassed to talk about.

MEDICAL MANAGEMENT

An enlarged prostate gland may be felt upon rectal digital examination and this remains a key diagnostic test. BPH can be managed in some men by conservative measures as the enlargement does not become too severe and symptomatic relief may be obtained with drug therapy (see below). The usual treatment of choice is surgery with transurethral resection of the prostate (TURP) being the main procedure employed. This operation involves introducing a cystoscope through the external urinary meatus which allows the surgeon to visualize the prostate. Using a cutting diathermy, he can then resect sufficient tissue to free the obstruction around the bladder neck and promote free drainage of urine. Such procedures do not require invasive surgery or general anaesthetics, which is very important as many patients are elderly. Closed irrigation of the bladder via an indwelling catheter postoperatively is crucial along with accurate fluid balance recording.

PHARMACOLOGY FOCUS

Reduction in the size of the prostate gland, sufficient to relieve symptoms in cases of moderate enlargement, occurs in response to lowered dihydrotestosterone levels. The drug finasteride inhibits the enzyme that transforms testosterone into the more potent form, dihydrotestosterone, and therefore helps men with less severe BPH.

Selective alpha-blocking drugs such as alfusozin produce smooth muscle relaxation in BPH and improve urinary flow rate as a result. They can also produce hypotension as an unwanted side effect, so patients should be carefully monitored if started on a course of one of these drugs.

PRIORITIES FOR NURSING CARE

Postoperatively:

1. Ensure that the catheter remains patent (a bladder irrigation system is usually set up) and drains freely as there is a risk of blocking by blood clots.

2. Accurate fluid balance ensures that there is no retention of urine or fluid overload, which could cause cardiac problems.
3. Vital sign monitoring as frequently as required to detect any cardiovascular or respiratory complications.
4. Ensure the patient's modesty and dignity at all times as many elderly men may find the whole postoperative period when they are catheterized very embarrassing.
5. Assist the patient to regain confidence and continence once the catheter is removed.
6. Explain procedures to the patient and family.
7. Remember that the patient's age means special attention has to be paid to the risk of pressure sores, DVT, chest infection, fluid intake and adequate nutrition. Early mobilization is therefore highly desirable.
8. Prevent cross-infection by care and attention to good technique when handling the catheter and drainage equipment.

PROSTATE CANCER (P776)

PATHOLOGY: Key facts

This is the second most common cause of mortality from malignant disease amongst men in the developed world, yet surprisingly little is known about the disorder. It is estimated that far more men die *with* cancer of the prostate than die *of* the disease, as it runs a lengthy and uncertain course mostly amongst older men. That said, it is responsible for the deaths of approximately 9500 men per year in the UK, 90% of whom are aged 65 or over.

WHAT TO LOOK OUT FOR

Initial symptoms are usually those encountered with BPH as the malignant growth in the gland interferes with the ability to void urine normally. The disease may not be discovered until far advanced and the man presents with a pathological fracture caused by metastatic spread to the skeleton.

MEDICAL MANAGEMENT

A great deal of controversy has surrounded testing for prostate specific antigen (PSA). Levels of this naturally occurring enzyme are frequently elevated (over 4 ng/mL) in cases of prostate cancer and this may be detected well before any clinical signs and symptoms are present. However, this test lacks sensitivity as some 20–30% of men with cancer of the prostate will not show an elevated reading and therefore be undetected by PSA alone. Worse, the test also lacks specificity and some 30–40% of those tested who show a positive PSA result do not actually have cancer as levels may be raised for a range of other reasons, including BPH. In primary care, clinicians are therefore strongly discouraged from ordering PSA tests as general screening for prostate cancer, even if men request the test because they have heard about it after reading a magazine or surfing on the net.

Medical treatment is problematic as no trials have shown any significant lengthening of life whether surgery to remove the prostate is performed (prostatectomy) or the patient is offered radiotherapy or chemotherapy. In fact, the risk of harm from treatment is the same as any chance of benefit.

PHARMACOLOGY FOCUS

In advanced prostate cancer where metastases are present, one of a group of drugs known as gonadorelin analogues may be used to deplete the body's androgen levels (buserelin or goserlin). Over a period of time, these drugs reduce the production of luteinizing hormone which in turn reduces androgen production.

PRIORITIES FOR NURSING CARE

The lack of any satisfactory preferred treatment for cancer of the prostate means that patient choice is particularly important. The nurse therefore has an important role in talking through the treatment options with the patient, including no treatment at all, to enable the patient to make his own decision. A great deal of psychological support will be needed. The man has to cope with the fact that he has a disease for which there is no proven effective treatment, and which could either be very aggressive and kill him inside a year, or with which he may live for many years, with relatively little trouble.

CHRONIC KIDNEY DISEASE AND RENAL FAILURE (P610)

Failure of kidney function leads to a build-up of waste products in the blood (uraemia) and has other serious metabolic consequences as homeostasis can no longer be maintained. This may occur as a sudden acute episode (acute renal failure), or as the final stage of chronic kidney disease (CKD) which is long-standing. Clinical signs of renal failure only become obvious when the kidneys have been reduced to working at only 25% of their capacity.

ACUTE RENAL FAILURE (P610)

PATHOLOGY: Key facts

There are many causes of acute renal failure (ARF) but they can be grouped into three main areas:

- *Prerenal*: caused by a reduced blood flow resulting in hypoperfusion of the kidney. This occurs secondary to serious hypovolaemia, hypotension or reduced cardiac output. ARF is therefore a major complication of shock.
- *Intrarenal*: produced by damage to the substance of the kidney commonly associated with acute tubular necrosis or toxic substances.
- *Postrenal*: conditions that obstruct the outflow of urine from the kidneys can cause the kidneys to fail, e.g. prostatic hyperplasia obstructing the outflow of urine from the bladder.

WHAT TO LOOK OUT FOR

The obvious initial sign is a reduction in urine output (oliguria) to below 35 mL/hour for the average size adult. If the cause is prerenal, signs of shock (hypotension, tachycardia, pale cold clammy skin, rapid respiration) will be obvious.

As ARF progresses the person becomes confused, and finally comatose, whilst pulmonary oedema will become more apparent.

MEDICAL MANAGEMENT

Blood chemistry is monitored very closely in order to assess the progress of the patient. Serum potassium is a very important measure as levels above normal increase the risk of a fatal cardiac arrhythmia. Fluid balance is crucial to prevent overloading the circulation with excess fluid leading to complications such as heart failure and pulmonary oedema. Dialysis will be necessary to maintain normal blood chemistry. Many patients with ARF begin to recover renal function within a few weeks if life-support measures (such as dialysis) enable them to survive the acute episode. The process of recovery is marked by a period of diuresis when urine output may rise to 4–5 L/day. Improvement in renal function may continue for several months.

PHARMACOLOGY FOCUS

Dangerously high potassium levels may be treated by an IVI of 50 mL glucose (50%) cation exchange resin and human soluble insulin or 10–20% glucose solution 4–6 hourly. This regime promotes the deposition of glucose as glycogen, a process that utilizes potassium and so reduces serum potassium levels. Intravenous fluids and medications will be prescribed in a complex regime that will be adjusted daily according to the patient's condition.

PRIORITIES FOR NURSING CARE

Patients in severe ARF are usually nursed in specialized units where the emphasis is on strict fluid/electrolyte balance and haemodialysis. Patient vital signs are closely monitored and great care taken to avoid sepsis arising from the increased vulnerability of ARF patients to infection. Diet is carefully controlled to reduce the intake of minerals such as sodium and potassium, as well as protein. Total parenteral nutrition may be necessary as the patient needs a high calorie intake, despite these restrictions.

CHRONIC KIDNEY DISEASE/RENAL FAILURE (P615)

PATHOLOGY: Key facts

Chronic kidney disease could be affecting as many as 1 in 10 mature adults. The kidneys still work, but their function, as measured by estimated glomerular filtration rate (eGFR) is deteriorating. It is now known to lead to complications such as an increased risk of cardiovascular disease, anaemia, bone disorders and hypertension. Hypertension makes the CKD worse and a positive feedback loop becomes established.

The eGFR is based upon serum creatinine. Creatinine is the metabolic byproduct of creatine, a small amino-acid-like molecule synthesized by the body as a source of ATP and therefore energy. It is produced at a constant rate, which only varies with body size (muscle mass). It is excreted in the urine by the kidneys, hence its basis as a measuring tool for GFR which is the amount of filtrate formed in all glomeruli in both kidneys per minute. The normal range is 120 ± 25 mL/min.1.73 m^2. CKD is classified into five types by falling eGFR. Type 5 equates to end stage renal failure in chronic renal failure (CRF). The patient has no symptoms in the early stages and may only be detected by an abnormal BP reading. In CRF the irreversible loss of function which affects the whole body will lead to death without treatment. Diabetes is the main cause.

WHAT TO LOOK OUT FOR

In the advanced stages of CKD when the patient is developing CRF:

- Fatigue, nausea, tiredness and generalized malaise caused by electrolyte and fluid balance disturbances, leading eventually to confusion and coma.
- Pale, dry, itchy skin with a yellowish tinge.
- Increased risk of infections, especially respiratory.
- Bone disorders (owing to disorder of calcium metabolism).
- Hypertension, cardiac arrhythmias.

- Gum sores and bleeding.
- Oedema.
- Gastrointestinal upsets and loss of appetite.

MEDICAL MANAGEMENT

The management of CKD aims at controlling contributing factors such as BP and blood sugar levels if diabetic. As end-stage renal failure develops (Stage 5 CKD) dialysis becomes inevitable. The best effective long-term treatment is transplantation but it may take many years before a suitable match with a donor kidney can be found.

Conservative treatment involves fluid and dietary restrictions aimed at preserving fluid and electrolyte balance. Fluid intake is restricted to match output whilst the diet involves restricting protein (approx 60 g/day) but increasing carbohydrate intake to provide adequate calories. The diet also has to be low in potassium, which excludes attractive foods such as chocolate, bananas and nuts.

Dialysis is instituted when conservative measures no longer keep blood chemistry within normal limits, e.g. when serum creatinine levels climb to around 800–1200 µmol/L. Two methods are used, one involving an external machine that purifies and returns blood to the body (haemodialysis) and the other that involves using the person's own peritoneum to filter out waste products (continual ambulatory peritoneal dialysis or CAPD).

The period of waiting for a donor kidney is a very difficult one for the patient as they struggle with a chronic and life-threatening disease that affects all aspects of their life. This is made worse by the knowledge that they are waiting for the death of another person to give them a kidney, which could transform their life but which may also be rejected by their own body, leaving them no better off. A great deal of psychological support is needed during this difficult period which may last for years.

PHARMACOLOGY FOCUS

Of particular concern are the serum calcium levels which may necessitate calcium supplements and vitamin D. Serum phosphate levels are controlled by the use of phosphate binders such as aluminium hydroxide whilst potassium exchange resins are prescribed if serum potassium levels are too high. Multivitamin tablets are also necessary as the person may become depleted of water-soluble vitamins. Contributory factors to CKD such as hypertension and diabetes need vigorous treatment and problems such as anaemia may also need drug therapy if significant.

PRIORITIES FOR NURSING CARE

Nurses play a crucial role in supporting the patient awaiting transplant both at home and during hospital visits. A great deal of education and encouragement is needed, paying particular attention to the following areas:

- Problems of depression and feelings of helplessness are common, requiring a great deal of support and understanding from the nurse for both patient and family.
- The patient and family should be taught to monitor fluid balance and what to look out for in terms of fluid overload or electrolyte imbalance (especially potassium).
- Dietary education and support.
- Decreased clotting ability in uraemic blood means that patient education about the potential for bleeding is required.
- Activity intolerance caused by anaemia and uraemia is common. A programme of gentle exercise negotiated with the patient helps.
- Skin and hair care are important due to the detrimental effects of uraemia on these tissues.
- Family members should be educated about the risk of a gradual clouding of consciousness which may develop as the tell-tale sign of increasing uraemia.

After transplant, the patient will be on a specialist unit where strict protocols will be followed to prevent rejection and infection secondary to the immunocompromised status of the patient.

TEN TOP TIPS

1. Always ensure that fluid balance charts are filled in accurately.
2. Check for the patency of catheter drainage, e.g. look out for kinks in the tubing.
3. Always wash your hands and wear gloves when handling catheters and drainage equipment.
4. Remember that patients may be very embarrassed by problems of incontinence.
5. Many causes of incontinence can be rectified.
6. The vast majority of people over 65 are continent.
7. Pelvic floor exercises are very effective in reducing stress incontinence.
8. CKD is a widespread disease and often a consequence of unhealthy lifestyles, it has a slow insidious onset and will only produce vague symptoms which the person would not normally associate with kidney disease at a late stage. Nursing observations such as elevated BP and abnormal findings on urine testing may be the first sign of CKD
9. Prevention of UTI is much more effective than treating it with antimicrobial medication.
10. Encourage regular fluid intake, particularly in older patients, to achieve set intake goals for each 24 hours.

8

Women's health

Anatomy at a glance   127
Physiology you need to know   129
Major conditions   130
Interruptions to pregnancy   130
Abortion   130
Ectopic pregnancy   133
Tumours of the ovary   134
Carcinoma of the cervix   135
Breast cancer   136
Ten top tips   141

ANATOMY AT A GLANCE

The female reproductive system may be divided into an external and an internal component.

The *external organs* have the collective name of the vulva, and are shown in Figure 8.1.

The *internal organs* consist of the

- *Vagina*: a tubular structure running backwards at an angle of 45 degrees to the vertical situated between the bladder and the rectum.
- *Uterus*: a hollow muscular organ which is shaped like a pear 7.5 cm long and 5 cm wide with relatively thick walls (2.5 cm). The cervix is that part of the uterus that protrudes into the vagina.
- *Uterine (Fallopian) tubes*: extend from the uterus towards the ovaries where they terminate in finger-like projections known as fimbriae which lie adjacent to the ovaries.
- *Ovaries*: each ovary is approximately 3 cm long and 2 cm wide. Surrounding the medulla is the cortex containing ovarian follicles in various stages of development, each of which contains an ovum.

The relationship of these organs is shown in Figure 8.2.

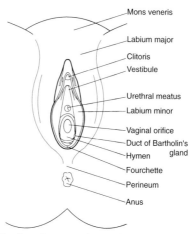

Figure 8.1 Female external genitalia.

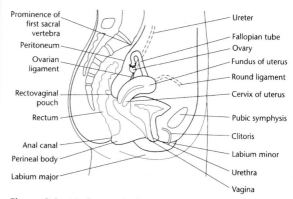

Figure 8.2 Median sagittal section of the female pelvis.

PHYSIOLOGY YOU NEED TO KNOW

The main functions of the female reproductive system are:

- To produce the female sex hormones oestrogen and progesterone.
- To ripen ova for fertilization.
- To facilitate the fertilization of ova.
- To incubate the fetus and deliver it into the outside world when it is ready to continue its growth and development as an infant.

Although at birth there are approximately two million oocytes present in the ovaries only 400–500 will develop to ovulation during adult life. Ovulation occurs when an ovarian follicle matures, ruptures and releases the ovum that it contains into the peritoneal cavity. Follicle-stimulating hormone (FSH) is responsible for the maturation process of the follicle (it also leads to the secretion of oestrogen, which stimulates the endometrium lining the uterus, preparing it for receiving a fertilized ovum). The anterior pituitary releases FSH, and it also releases another hormone known as luteinizing hormone (LH), which stimulates the cells lining the follicle (after ovulation) to develop into the corpus luteum. This will produce progesterone.

Two fates may befall the ovum. If it is fertilized it embeds itself in the wall of the uterus where it continues to develop, producing human chorionic gonadotrophin in the process. This hormone continues to stimulate the corpus luteum to produce progesterone for the first three months of the pregnancy. If the ovum is not fertilized, the corpus luteum decays and a new menstrual cycle will commence about 14 days after ovulation with menstruation.

Reproductive function ceases at around age 50, the menopause, when menstruation stops. On average, therefore, women live for some 30 years in this post-menopausal state. The menopause is a time in a woman's life when her hormonal balance is severely disrupted as oestrogen levels fall dramatically. Hot flushes are one very pronounced symptom associated with low oestrogen levels and pulses of LH. The woman experiences acute physical discomfort as she feels very hot and her skin reddens, particularly around the face and neck. Episodes are unpredictable and sudden in onset, although they gradually decline in frequency as the now postmenopausal hormonal balance is established.

MAJOR CONDITIONS

There are many health problems related to the female reproductive tract. This chapter concentrates only on those that account for the maximum amount of treatment required, particularly as in-patients. You are encouraged to read and study much further afield to understand the full picture of women's health. Do remember the sociological dimension to women's health, and how women's role in society plays such a big part in determining health.

INTERRUPTIONS TO PREGNANCY (P797)

ABORTION

PATHOLOGY: Key facts

Abortion is defined as the cessation of pregnancy before the 24th week of pregnancy. This can occur spontaneously or may be induced for therapeutic reasons. Spontaneous abortion usually results from:

- Problems with the fetus due to chromosomal or developmental abnormalities which are incompatible with life.
- Maternal problems such as a severe infection of the mother, side effects of drugs or hormonal imbalances.
- Environmental factors such as trauma or nutritional deficits affecting the mother.

Therapeutic abortion is performed for either medical or social reasons, and is controlled by legislation in the UK and many other countries. Despite this, criminal abortions are still performed, which can have disastrous consequences for the woman.

WHAT TO LOOK OUT FOR

Vaginal bleeding during pregnancy is abnormal and the woman should be seen by a midwife or doctor immediately as this may indicate a threatened abortion. At this stage it is still possible to save the pregnancy. Severe bleeding and pain usually indicate that an inevitable abortion has occurred, however, and the pregnancy cannot be saved.

Sometimes the woman experiences a missed abortion, in which there may be a brownish discharge early in the pregnancy accompanied by a weak pregnancy test. The classic early symptoms of pregnancy may have ceased sooner than expected. The obstetrican will usually evacuate the remains of the pregnancy about 2 weeks after the estimated death of the fetus. This eliminates the risk of disseminated intravascular coagulation, and reduces the distress the woman probably experiences from knowing that she is carrying the remains of her dead fetus within the uterus.

MEDICAL MANAGEMENT

Retained products of conception pose a major infection hazard; therefore, after inevitable abortion, such products must be fully removed. This may have to be done as an emergency procedure on the ward using swabs, sponges and forceps with a speculum. In less urgent situations, dilation of the cervix and evacuation of the uterus may be performed. All products of conception should be saved for histology.

Therapeutic abortions may be performed surgically by suction, dilatation and curettage as a day case. They are best performed before 12–14 weeks of gestation. Alternatively, a medical abortion may be induced by giving a single 600 mg oral dose of mifepristone followed by 1 mg of gemeprost (a prostaglandin preparation) by vagina. This is most effective in the first 9 weeks of pregnancy.

Later terminations, after 12–14 weeks, require different techniques. Prostaglandins may be given IV, regulated by infusion pump to induce labour. The fetus dies and is expelled with assistance of oxytocin. Alternatively, gemeprost can be given as a vaginal pessary 1 mg every 3 hours to induce a late abortion (maximum dose 5 mg) after treatment with mifepristone.

PHARMACOLOGICAL FOCUS

Mifepristone is an anti-progesterone agent. A pregnancy requires progesterone to prevent uterine contractions, therefore reducing progesterone levels makes it easier to induce uterine contractions with prostaglandins, and so expel the fetus.

PRIORITIES FOR NURSING CARE

If the woman has a threatened abortion, rest and close observation are essential. It will be a very anxious time, and a lot of support is needed to help the woman cope with the fear of possibly losing her pregnancy.

If a therapeutic abortion is carried out, or the abortion becomes inevitable, the patient needs close observation and regular monitoring of vital signs. The abortion may well involve labour pains that will be particularly distressing to the woman. Analgesia and support are essential. Patient education prior to discharge is a vital nursing role, concentrating on the following key points:

- Resume normal activity gradually.
- Intermittent menstrual-like discharge is to be expected for the next 2 weeks but it should not be bright red in colour; sanitary pads should be used. She should abstain from sexual intercourse while the discharge is present.
- Some cramping is to be expected, but severe discomfort or fever should be reported immediately to the doctor.
- A menstrual period is to be expected 4–5 weeks after abortion.
- Information concerning a follow-up appointment and how to obtain support and counselling.

An abortion will mean different things to different women. To many it is a distressing experience and a great deal of help and psychological support is needed to help the woman through this difficult period in her life. Family planning advice may also be indicated, depending upon the circumstances surrounding the pregnancy and its termination.

ECTOPIC PREGNANCY (P796)

PATHOLOGY: Key facts

Ectopic pregnancy occurs when a fertilized ovum is implanted anywhere outside the uterus. It usually occurs in the Fallopian tube when passage of the zygote has been impeded. The incidence of ectopic pregnancy seems to have been increasing over the last 15 years, and this is thought to be associated with factors such as increased rates of pelvic infection, widespread use of intra-uterine devices (IUDs), or fertility induced by ovulatory agents. Usually, the fetus dies as the chorionic villi burrow into the tubal wall and rupture a blood vessel leading to bleeding. Occasionally, the tube may be ruptured.

WHAT TO LOOK OUT FOR

The woman will have the signs of early pregnancy, and may not have had a period for 6–10 weeks. The history is one of localized abdominal pain on one side, which becomes sharper and intermittent (due to waves of peristalsis in the tube attempting to pass the embryo or abortus). Finally there is usually a short episode of severe localized pain as the embryo finally separates from the tube wall, followed by generalized abdominal pain. Occasionally, the woman experiences acute and severe abdominal pain followed by nausea, vomiting and vaginal bleeding, indicating a ruptured fallopian tube. This is followed by signs of shock and collapse resulting from severe internal bleeding.

MEDICAL MANAGEMENT

Diagnosis of an ectopic pregnancy usually depends upon a single pregnancy test, or serial ones, ultrasonography and if necessary laparoscopy. If a ruptured tubal pregnancy is suspected, the woman will need urgent surgery for removal of the Fallopian tube and fetus (salpingectomy).

PRIORITIES FOR NURSING CARE

Close observation and monitoring of vital signs is essential. A great deal of psychological support will be needed.

TUMOURS OF THE OVARY (P811)

PATHOLOGY: Key facts

Tumours may be non-malignant and consist of cysts which expand as more fluid accumulates. Ovarian cysts such as these are seen during the reproductive years. Polycystic disease of the ovary occurs in the early 20s, and is caused by an endocrine imbalance leading to the ovaries producing an excessive amount of androgens. Sterility, hirsutism and secondary amenorrhoea may follow. Ovarian tumours can also be malignant. Pseudomucinous cystadenomas are the most common neoplasms of the ovary. They may become bilateral and malignant as may serous cystadenomas. Dermoid cysts are rarely malignant, however. A cancer in one ovary may quickly spread to the other because of the close lymphatic connections. Approximately 5% of all female cancers arise in the ovary.

WHAT TO LOOK OUT FOR

Initially an ovarian tumour produces no noticeable symptoms. However, as it enlarges it compresses the bladder leading to frequency of micturition. Growth in size of the tumour leads to constipation, oedema of the legs, anorexia and a feeling of fullness. Ascites may develop, interfering with breathing, and pain gradually develops as tissue become further stretched and compressed by the tumour.

MEDICAL MANAGEMENT

The risk of malignant changes means that ovarian tumours are watched carefully by doctors with biopsy and laparotomy performed early. Surgical resection of the tumour is indicated if it is benign, but total hysterectomy and bilateral salpingo-oophorectomy (removal of the uterus and Fallopian tubes) is carried out in cases of malignancy. Chemotherapy follows surgery, but survival rates are poor as many tumours have metastasized before discovery. Treatment is often palliative, and directed towards symptom relief such as paracentesis for ascites.

PRIORITIES FOR NURSING CARE

If the patient has surgery for a malignant tumour (hysterectomy), she will need intensive postoperative care for any major surgery. Thromboemboli are a particular risk for such patients and every care should be taken to prevent them with early ambulation, leg exercises, TED stockings and deep breathing exercises.

CARCINOMA OF THE CERVIX (P812)

PATHOLOGY: Key facts

Risk factors include infection with certain strains of the human papillomavirus, smoking and beginning sexual activity young with multiple partners. The disease is preceded by changes in cells (dysplasia) at the squamocolumnar junction of the cervix, which may be detected by histology. Some of the early changes detected may be reversible and do not automatically mean that the woman will develop cancer. If changes have progressed to the point where a cancer in situ is said to be present (Stage 0), it is estimated that within 10 years 50% of such women will have invasive cancer (Stage I). Such invasive cancers spread to other structures nearby (Stage II), and then the pelvic walls and lower vagina (Stage III). In advanced disease (Stage IV), the bladder and bowel are involved and distant metastases may be present. Cervical smears offer the best chance of detecting premalignant changes before carcinoma in situ has developed. Treatment at this early stage leads to very good results.

WHAT TO LOOK OUT FOR

The woman has no symptoms initially but eventually may develop some vaginal bleeding or an unusual discharge with an offensive odour. Pain is a late sign, and when accompanied by anorexia and weight loss indicates that the disease is already well advanced.

MEDICAL MANAGEMENT

If definite changes in cells (dysplasia) are present, a punch biopsy is performed to allow detailed inspection of tissue.

Cervical dysplasia may be treated by diathermy excision (LLETZ, Large Loop Excision of the Transformational Zone, or LEEP, Loop Electrical Excision Procedure) as may more-extensive lesions, but then a general anaesthetic is required. Cryotherapy (freezing of the transformational zone) is an alternative for cervical dysplasia. A cone biopsy removes a cone-shaped section of the central cervix, which on examination may contain all of the malignant tissue. The biopsy is then considered sufficient treatment. If invasive cancer is found, it will be treated according to the stage at which it has been found.

PRIORITIES FOR NURSING CARE

Hysterectomy is a major surgical procedure, and the woman will require intensive nursing care to help her recover physically from the operation. There are the additional factors of how she may feel about herself as a woman having lost her uterus and other reproductive organs. A great deal of understanding and psychological support is needed, in addition to the standard nursing care required after surgery.

BREAST CANCER (P817)

PATHOLOGY: Key facts

Breast cancer is the most common cancer in women world-wide and in the UK, over 40,000 women are diagnosed with the condition each year. In some families breast cancer is hereditary, and two genes (BRCA1 and BRCA2) have now been identified that confer the disease risk on descendants. Other risk factors include:

- Early menarche (before age 12).
- Late menopause (over 55).
- Age; most breast cancers occur in older women.
- Not having borne children (nulliparous).
- Having a first child at over 35 years of age.
- Obesity.

■ Long-term use of hormone replacement therapy is associated with a slight increase in absolute risk.

WHAT TO LOOK OUT FOR

The following signs are most significant:

■ The woman has usually found a lump in her breast herself. However, this may be a benign cyst rather than a cancer. In fact, some 90% of breast lumps that women report are *not* cancer. A cancer can occur anywhere in the breast but the most likely site is the upper outer quadrant (50% of cancers), whilst the lower outer quadrant is the least likely (6%).
■ Nipple discharge.
■ Nodularity or thickening of tissue in one specific area.
■ A breast that appears to have enlarged.
■ Dimpled or creased appearance in the breast.

Breast awareness is taught to women. This involves regularly looking at both breasts and feeling them using the flat part of the fingers (not the palms). This should not be performed just before a period is due, however, as there will be menstrual-related changes occurring which confuse the picture. The woman should be looking for any changes that have occurred. There is little evidence this actually leads to early detection or improves long-term survival.

MEDICAL MANAGEMENT

Diagnostic investigations include:

■ *Mammography (breast X-ray).* The NHS screening programme aims to screen all women between 50–70 years of age. However, there is considerable debate whether this programme improves survival rates amongst women as early detection of a cancer does not improve the prognosis.
■ *Ultrasonography* is more useful in younger women as the increased breast tissue density in younger women limits the diagnostic value of the X-rays that may be obtained by mammography.

■ *Cytology.* The fine-needle aspiration cytology technique allows a rapid diagnosis to be made. Alternative breast biopsy techniques such as the Tru-cut or Advanced Breast Biopsy Instrumentation System may be used.

Surgery is the definitive first line of treatment but a range of procedures are available. The surgeon has to consider factors such as the stage of the cancer, its size and the size of the woman's breast before recommending a procedure which could involve removal of

■ The whole breast (mastectomy).
■ The breast plus surrounding tissue and lymphatic tissue (modified radical mastectomy).
■ The breast lump only (lumpectomy).
■ The lump plus the breast quadrant involved (quadrantectomy).

After lumpectomy or quadrantectomy the surviving breast tissue is irradiated as a precaution. This may be done by radioactive implants or external beam radiotherapy. Whatever the surgical procedure, reconstructive surgery may be offered to the woman, involving a breast implant, for example.

The woman will be considered for drug therapy and chemotherapy after surgery because of the risk of metastases already having spread to other parts of the body.

Unfortunately, owing to fear and embarrassment, some women still present with a fungating advanced breast cancer that is inoperable. In such cases, radiotherapy and chemotherapy are offered as palliative treatment.

PHARMACOLOGY FOCUS

Many breast cancers are sensitive to hormonal manipulation. This has led to the development of tamoxifen as a very important drug in treating breast cancer. It acts as an antagonist at oestrogen receptor sites and is therefore very effective against oestrogen receptor-positive breast cancers (i.e. cancers that respond to oestrogens). It has been shown to delay the growth of metastases and increase survival whilst it is also beneficial in the treatment of established metastatic disease. Chemotherapy may be given in addition to tamoxifen in carefully selected cases.

PRIORITIES FOR NURSING CARE

After Surgery

In addition to normal postoperative care, attention should be paid to the following:

- Drains from the wound should be carefully checked and removed at 24–48 hrs.
- Axillary drains should stay until they have stopped draining serosanguinous fluid, which may be several days.
- Careful observation for the development of a haematoma (accumulation of blood) or seroma (accumulation of serous fluid beneath the wound) is necessary despite the drains which have been sited to try and prevent these potential complications.
- Encouragement with physiotherapy and arm exercises which start 24 hours postoperatively. These are essential if the patient is to recover a good range of movement in the arm.
- The patient should be encouraged to look at the wound whilst still in hospital. This can be very traumatic but is a step that has to be taken. A great deal of support and understanding will be needed to help the woman come to terms with her radically altered self-image.
- A breast-care specialist nurse will normally visit the woman and if she has had a mastectomy, arrange for her to have a soft breast form fitted into a supportive bra before she is discharged. This will give her a reasonably natural appearance in the short term, whilst long-term options are considered.
- Discussions should take place concerning the long-term complications such as secondary lymphoedema arising from disruption of the normal lymphatic drainage caused by surgery and radiotherapy. The woman may notice painful swelling of the arm on the affected side many months later. Measurement of arm circumference provides useful baseline data for future comparison, and a range of exercises can be taught to help promote lymphatic drainage.

After Radiotherapy (p208)

■ Localized skin reactions occur leading to erythema, swelling and soreness of the breast. In such cases no topical applications should be applied other than topical hydrocortisone 1%. Skin breakdown may occur in which case radiation therapy is stopped until the skin recovers.

■ Psychological effects such as depression and tiredness are common, especially as the woman may be travelling long distances to attend as a day patient for her therapy and her home life may be difficult.

■ Nausea and hair loss are *not* associated with localized radiotherapy, however.

After Chemotherapy (p198)

■ Adjuvant breast chemotherapy regimes tend to cause less hair loss than other regimes; however, significant thinning may still occur. Scalp cooling may reduce the amount of hair loss.

■ Some agents cause sore and sticky eyes which may be treated with artificial tears or folinic acid.

■ A sore mouth is common. Oral hygiene should be encouraged, including the use of a soft toothbrush, along with a good fluid intake (2.5 L/day).

■ Herpes simplex ulcers may develop and should be treated promptly with aciclovir.

■ A good well-balanced diet is essential to aid recovery from chemotherapy.

■ Nausea and vomiting are major problems. Anti-emetic drugs should be administered and the woman may find eating small meals more frequently is helpful.

■ A lowered blood count may develop as a result of the harmful effects of the chemotherapy on developing blood cells in the bone marrow. Any unusual tendency to bruising (low platelet count) or recurring infections (low white cell count) or feeling of tiredness (anaemia due to low red cell count) should be reported at once. Frequent bloods should be taken to monitor the blood count picture.

■ Diarrhoea can develop as a result of chemotherapy damaging the cells lining the gastrointestinal mucosa. Anti-diarrhoeal drugs may help.

■ Lethargy is a major problem affecting women towards the end of their chemotherapy regime and they should be reassured that this is a normal side effect.

Metastatic Disease

Unfortunately, breast cancer can spread to involve the skeleton, lungs, liver, brain and other tissues of the body. Careful follow-up of the patient is therefore essential after initial treatment. Should metastatic disease occur, the focus of treatment is on palliation rather than cure.

TEN TOP TIPS

1. The psychological impact of procedures such as mastectomy or hysterectomy can be devastating on the woman. A great deal of psychological support is needed.
2. Reflect upon how you would feel as a woman if you had to undergo such a procedure.
3. Also consider the impact upon the family – her husband/partner may find it very difficult to come to terms with the alteration in body image involved.
4. There is a great deal of controversy about the effectiveness of breast self-awareness and breast screening programmes. Women will turn to you as a nurse for answers to these questions, so keep yourself up to date with the latest evidence, research and policy debates.
5. Use health education opportunities to encourage attendance for cervical screening.
6. Encourage safer sex, especially with younger women and teenagers, who are the group most at risk for sexually transmitted infections such as *Chlamydia*.
7. Make younger women aware of the potential for asymptomatic sexually transmitted infections and the long-term risks of pelvic inflammatory disease that can occur as a result, such as sterility and ectopic pregnancy.

8. Remind women that HIV/AIDS is also a problem for heterosexual women.

9. Be aware that the loss of a pregnancy is a very personal thing to a woman, it means different things to different women.

10. A woman's reaction to a diagnosis of cancer is rarely predictable, and can range from a determination to fight the disease to the very last, to total devastation and despair.

9

Caring for the patient with a disorder of the nervous system

Anatomy at a glance   143
Physiology you need to know   148
Cerebrovascular accident (CVA)   149
Head injury   154
Brain tumours   159
Degenerative disorders of the nervous system   162
Ten top tips   164

ANATOMY AT A GLANCE (P653)

The nervous system is structurally composed of two parts, the central nervous system (brain, cranial nerves and spinal cord) and the peripheral nervous system, which consists of the spinal nerves connecting to the rest of the body.

If the nervous system is considered in terms of its function, it can again be split into two parts:

■ The somatic (voluntary) nervous system which transmits messages to and from the non-visceral part of the body (skeletal, skin, etc.), and is generally under conscious control.
■ The autonomic nervous system which is concerned with the regulation of visceral muscles and glands and as such is not usually under conscious control.

The nervous system consists of two main groups of cells, neurones and neuroglia.

Neurones
These are the functional cells responsible for initiating or transmitting messages (see Figure 9.1). Each neurone has a

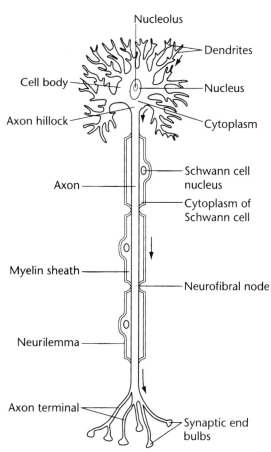

Figure 9.1 Structure of a typical neurone.

nucleus, one or more projections known as dendrites, which conduct the nerve impulse *into* the cell body, and a single long projection known as an axon, which conducts the nerve impulse *away* from the cell body to the next cell. Cell bodies are generally known as grey matter, while axons make up the white matter. Where the axon of one neurone meets the dendrite of the next, a synapse is said to occur. Although the axon and dendrite of the two neurones are in close proximity, they are not connected. The nerve impulse is transmitted via neurotransmitter molecules which cross the synapse. Neurones can have a sensory, motor or connecting function (interneurones).

Neuroglia

These are supportive and protective cells. They make up approximately 50% of the volume of the CNS, and are divided into different types depending upon their specialist functions. Unlike neurones, they can divide and multiply but they cannot pass messages.

The Central Nervous System

The brain is what makes us human through its ability for thought, consciousness and intelligence. It is also responsible for controlling motor function, receiving and interpreting sensory input and regulation of the whole body environment through the autonomic nervous system and by interacting with the endocrine system. The higher functions of the brain are concentrated in the cerebrum. Other important parts of the brain are summarized below:

- *Basal ganglia* are groups of nerve cells deeply imbedded within the white matter whose function is not clearly understood.
- *Thalami* (singular thalamus) are relay stations for sensory messages incoming to the brain.
- *Hypothalamus* contains important centres to do with temperature regulation, hunger, thirst and emotion. It is also responsible for controlling much endocrine function via its association with the pituitary gland.
- *Brainstem* consists of three portions
  - The medulla oblongata consists of ascending and descending nerve pathways, and contains vital autonomic centres controlling breathing, heart rate, and vasomotor tone as well as centres controlling the following reflexes: vomiting, coughing, sneezing and gagging.
  - The pons Varolii consists of many nerve tracts linking the medulla with the upper portion of the brainstem, the midbrain (pons means bridge in Latin).

- The midbrain contains grey matter (nucleii) and white matter (axons) and is the site of the cerebral aqueduct which connects the 3rd and 4th ventricles.

■ *Ventricles.* These consist of four cavities through which the cerebrospinal fluid circulates.

■ *Cerebrospinal fluid (CSF).* This fluid bathes the whole brain and spinal cord. The average adult has 125–150 ml of CSF which is a clear water-like liquid. It circulates via the subarachnoid space and cerebral aqueducts acting as a shock absorber for the brain.

■ *Meninges.* These are the three outer layers that cover the brain and spinal cord. The tough fibrous outer layer is known as the dura mater, the middle layer is the arachnoid mater and the very delicate inner layer is the pia mater. The space between the arachnoid and pia mater (subarachnoid space) is full of CSF.

■ *Spinal cord.* This originates at the medulla oblongata, running down within the vertebral column to the level of the first or second lumbar vertebra. Spinal nerves exit and join at each space between the vertebrae. The remaining nerves exit the vertebral column at the level of the intervertebral disc which separates L1 and L2 to form a delicate fan-like structure known as the cauda equina. Within the spinal cord are both grey matter (neuronal cell bodies) and major nerve trunks (axons) conveying messages to and from the brain via sensory and motor pathways.

Blood Supply to the Brain

The brain receives approximately 20% of cardiac output and consumes 20% of all the oxygen that the body uses. As the brain has no reserve stores of glucose or oxygen, any reduction in blood supply will have immediate and serious effects. Brain cells suffer irreversible damage within 2–4 minutes of losing their blood supply.

The blood supply to the brain is derived from the two internal carotid arteries and two vertebral arteries which unite to form the basilar artery. Various small connecting arteries link these two arterial systems to form what is known collectively as the circle of Willis.

Cranial Nerves

The 12 pairs of *cranial nerves* are conventionally numbered in Roman numerals from I to XII. Cranial nerves III through XII emerge from the brainstem, whilst I and II are purely sensory and are directly connected to the appropriate sensory centre in the brain (I is olfactory and II is the optic nerve). The Xth cranial nerve is the vagus nerve, and its motor branch is part of the autonomic nervous system which is responsible for regulating smooth muscle function in a wide range of visceral organs.

Spinal Nerves

There are 31 pairs of spinal nerves arising from the spinal cord. They are described as mixed because they contain both motor and sensory nerve fibres. The motor fibres exit the spinal cord at the front (anterior root), whilst sensory input to the spinal cord is via the posterior root.

The Autonomic Nervous System

This contains both sensory and motor nerves and controls the visceral function of the body affecting everything from heart rate, diameter of blood vessels (and hence blood pressure) through to gastrointestinal function. There are two divisions of the autonomic nervous system:

- *The Sympathetic Nervous System*: this originates in the lumbar and thoracic regions of the spinal cord and produces generalized responses that help the body cope with threat and stress known as the 'fight or flight response'. These include, for example, bronchodilation and increasing heart rate.
- *The Parasympathetic Nervous System*: approximately 75% of all parasympathetic fibres travel in the vagus nerve (Xth cranial). Parasympathetic nerves promote a state of resting and conservation of body resources whilst eliminating waste.

Generally speaking, both the sympathetic and parasympathetic systems innervate the same organs but have opposing effects. As a simplification, it may help to think of the sympathetic division as acting like the accelerator pedal of a car, whilst the parasympathetic division acts as the brake.

PHYSIOLOGY YOU NEED TO KNOW

Nerve impulse transmission depends upon the following series of events:

1. A resting neurone is in a polarized state. As a result the outside of the neurone carries a positive charge and the inside a negative charge.
2. A stimulus causes a localized alteration in the permeability of the nerve cell membrane resulting in the movement of large numbers of positively charged sodium ions into the cell.
3. The outer part of the membrane now has a negative charge and the inside of the neurone acquires a positive charge. Depolarization of this portion of the cell membrane has occurred and this triggers voltage-gated ion channels in the next section of the axon to open allowing more positive sodium ions to rush into the axon triggering further depolarization.
4. This zone of depolarization now sweeps down the length of the axon, followed by repolarization of the cell membrane as it reverts to its original state. This change in polarity is referred to as an action potential.
5. When the action potential reaches the end of the nerve axon, it stimulates the release of various molecules known as neurotransmitters.
6. Neurotransmitter molecules move from the end of the axon across the gap to the next neurone in the chain. This gap is known as a synapse. The next cell may be a muscle cell, which is being stimulated by a motor neurone to contract, in which case this is known as a neuromuscular junction.
7. The neurotransmitter molecules lock onto specific receptor sites on the membrane of the next nerve or muscle cell (postsynaptic membrane) where their presence may initiate a new wave of depolarization (action potential) to spread through the next neurone and on to the next axon in the chain.
   - The speed with which nerve impulses are conducted in this way increases with the width of the axon conduct-

ing the impulse and also is greatly increased by the presence of a myelin sheath surrounding the axon.

● Nerves are *not* in contact with each other at a synapse. The gap is referred to as the synaptic cleft.

● Some neurotransmitters act to block the transmission of an impulse (inhibitory neurotransmitters).

● Some molecules can act as hormones and neurotransmitters such as epinephrine (adrenaline).

● Many drugs work by blocking the effect of neurotransmitters (such as beta blockers) or by imitating this effect in a controlled therapeutic way in order to achieve an enhanced effect (such as salbutamol).

CEREBROVASCULAR ACCIDENT (CVA) [P672]

PATHOLOGY: Key facts

A CVA involves an interruption of the blood supply to a part of the brain and the consequent development of neurological deficits which can be mild to severe and in extreme cases fatal. The cause of the interruption can be:

■ Atherosclerosis which narrows and gradually occludes the lumen of one of the cerebral arteries.

■ A thrombosis associated with atherosclerosis of the carotid, vertebral or other cerebral artery.

■ An embolism, usually derived from a cerebral thrombosis, may lodge in an artery and block it.

■ A rupture of the cerebral artery wall (associated with atherosclerosis and/or hypertension).

Additionally, many patients suffer transient ischaemic attacks (TIA) before a major CVA. These TIAs occur when disease of the arterial wall leads to a temporary reduction in blood supply, and they are an early warning sign of serious problems ahead. They typically last only a few minutes or a few hours and the neurological deficit they produce resolves spontaneously (e.g. slurred speech, visual disturbances, paresis, dizziness, confusion). Eighty per cent of people who have a thrombotic stroke have had preceding TIAs.

Most CVAs occur in people aged over 60. However, a significant number occur in young adults when the cause is a congenital weakness in a cerebral artery known as a cerebral aneurysm. The person is born with a weak area lacking muscle and elastic tissue in one of their cerebral arteries. Gradually over the years, this protrudes as a swelling from the arterial wall (hence the common name berry aneurysm), which may then start to leak or in worst cases, rupture completely, which is usually fatal. The bleeding may be into the subarachnoid space (subarachnoid haemorrhage) or into the brain substance itself.

Commonly there is a volume of oedematous tissue around the damaged region and as a result of raised intracranial pressure, neuronal function decreases. The extent of this oedema peaks at around 72 hours. It is only when this oedema has resolved over the next 2 weeks or so that the full extent of the patient's functional loss can be estimated.

WHAT TO LOOK OUT FOR

- Level of consciousness is the key observation for all neurological patients whether they have had a CVA, head injury or any other neurological disorder. Any deterioration in their condition will usually show itself by a decrease in the level of consciousness. This is assessed objectively by the Glasgow Coma Scale (GCS) (see Table 9.1), and these observations may be carried out as frequently as every 15 minutes in an unstable patient. The GCS is based upon the *best* responses to objective measures of how awake the patient is (eye opening), motor ability and how oriented they are (verbal responses).
- Vital signs. Rising intracranial pressure leads to an increase in blood pressure as the heart works harder to supply blood to the brain. A reflex slowing of pulse rate may also occur as blood pressure rises. This is a relatively late sign of rising intracranial pressure and neurological disorder; diminished level of consciousness will have preceded this observation. Disturbance to both the rate and rhythm of respiration can occur as a result of a CVA, especially if it involves the brainstem, therefore

Table 9.1 The Glasgow Coma Scale

Eye opening	Spontaneous	4 points
	To speech	3 points
	To pain	2 points
	None	1 point
Motor response	Obeys command	6 points
	Localizes	5 points
	Flexion	4 points
	Abnormal flexion	3 points
	Extension	2 points
	None	1 point
Verbal response	Oriented	5 points
	Confused	4 points
	Inappropriate words	3 points
	Incomprehensible sounds	2 points
	None	1 point

respiratory rate and rhythm should be carefully monitored.

■ Limb weakness (hemiplegia) is a common sign of a CVA. Assess strength of the arms by asking the patient to hold them out level in front of them. Strength of the legs can be assessed by pressing against the soles of the patient's feet, whilst they are lying down, and asking them to push you away by extending the feet downwards.

■ Pupil reflexes are checked in most patients with neurological disorder. Rising intracranial pressure leads to compression of cranial nerve III (oculomotor) which innervates the iris. As a result the pupil becomes sluggish to respond to light, the pupil dilates and in the worst case becomes fixed and dilated. This can occur on one side only indicating a localized lesion such as a haematoma is compressing the oculomotor nerve on that side only, or if both pupils are affected this suggests a generalized increase in intracranial pressure. Diminishing level of consciousness usually occurs *before* changing pupil reflexes.

■ Other important neurological signs that should be reported immediately include headaches, vomiting, photophobia, any visual disturbances and convulsions.

MEDICAL MANAGEMENT

Diagnosis is crucial and after a thorough clinical examination, medical staff may order several diagnostic tests:

■ Skull/spinal radiography.
■ Computed tomography (CT) scan to produce a series of detailed cross-sectional brain images.
■ Magnetic resonance imaging (MRI) scan also produces detailed brain images which are better for investigating some areas (e.g. spinal cord).
■ Carotid Doppler Ultrasonography assesses the blood flow to the brain through the carotid arteries.
■ Electroencephalogram (EEG) permits study of the electrical activity of the brain which is recorded as a characteristic series of wave patterns.
■ Lumbar puncture involves the insertion of a spinal needle between the 3rd/4th or 4th/5th lumbar vertebrae into the subarachnoid space around the spinal cord. This allows an estimate to be made of lumbar CSF pressure and samples of CSF to be withdrawn for analysis. The procedure is contraindicated if intracranial pressure is raised, however, as damage to the brain may occur as a result of the sudden change in pressure that will occur.

After diagnosis, medical management of stroke patients is usually conservative and symptomatic. However, patients who survive a subarachnoid haemorrhage will be considered for surgery to clip the aneurysm in order to prevent a re-bleed. Surgery may also be considered for patients experiencing TIAs. The operation aims to remove atheroma from the intima of the internal carotid artery (endarterectomy) and strengthen the wall of the artery with a dacron graft in order to avoid a full scale CVA.

PRIORITIES FOR NURSING CARE

■ Close observation of level of consciousness and vital signs because of risk of further stroke developing.
■ Assessment of pressure areas and a pressure sore prevention regime of regular turning plus the use of pressure-relieving devices.

- Fluid balance must be carefully monitored with a set volume of intake per 24 hours. Initially this may be restricted to reduce the risk of cerebral oedema and raised intracranial pressure. Output should also be accurately monitored, although incontinence is a common problem.

- Soft diet is encouraged as soon as practicable, depending upon the patient's ability to swallow. Laxatives may be required to prevent constipation although faecal incontinence can also occur due to loss of the defecation reflex.

- The potential for injury is large because of confusion and impaired motor skills. Close observation is therefore essential and cot sides should be managed according to local policy.

- Teamwork with the physiotherapists is essential to give the patient the best chance of recovering some function and avoiding the development of painful contractures in affected limbs.

- Assistance with all aspects of personal hygiene is essential, especially the mouth and eyes.

- Sensory deficits after the stroke may leave the patient prone to developing burns or other lesions. The patient may have impaired vision. Proprioception deficit means the patient is now unaware of the relative positions of different parts of the body.

- Speech disturbance (aphasia) may occur, which is very frustrating for the patient and requires a great deal of understanding from the nurse.

- Psychological support is a major factor in helping the patient and family come to terms with what has happened. Unrealistic promises of recovery must be avoided at all costs. However, the patient may become very anxious, depressed or angry at their disability and need a great deal of understanding and encouragement to promote optimal rehabilitation.

- Major social changes may follow as the person may be unable to return to their previous home and lifestyle as a consequence of their disabilities. Social isolation is another major potential problem.

- The recovery and rehabilitation process is a true multi-disciplinary effort and takes a lengthy period of time. A great deal of teaching for both patient and family is required including relearning skills that were originally learned a lifetime ago. The nursing staff, both hospital and community based, have to contribute fully to the work of the multidisciplinary team (MDT). Ongoing care from the District Nursing service can give the patient a high degree of independence in the community as part of the MDT effort. The degree of functional deficit can only be reliably estimated some 2 weeks after the stroke (see Pathology above).

HEAD INJURY (P683)

PATHOLOGY: Key facts

Intracranial pressure (ICP) is the pressure exerted by CSF within the ventricles of the brain (normally 0–15 mmHg). One of the main features of head injury is an increase in ICP, which in turn causes compromised blood supply to the brain (cerebral ischaemia), and hence brain damage. It can also cause displacement of brain tissue or CSF. The ICP is usually elevated either as a direct result of trauma to brain tissue (swelling accompanies injury in most areas of the body), or the formation of a haematoma from a torn blood vessel.

Head injury may be associated with a skull fracture which may be open, allowing potential contamination and infection to complicate the injury. If the skull fracture is depressed this may also lead to an increased risk of convulsions. A fracture through the base of the skull is also considered to be open as it allows communication between the oropharynx and the meninges, leading to the risk of meningitis.

Less-severe head injuries are known as concussion injury and are characterized by a jarring effect on the brain and its sudden contact with the inside of the skull. There may be a short period of unconsciousness of up to a few minutes but the primary brain injury is mild. Upon regaining concsciousness the person may be slightly dazed and confused, complaining of headache and have a slight period of amnesia.

More severe injuries involving greater force lead to cerebral contusion (bruising) and laceration. The patient may lose consciousness for a lengthy period of time and severe primary brain injury may occur. A serious possibility is the patient who suffers a short period of unconsciousness and then regains consciousness, appearing to have recovered (the lucid interval) before suffering a decline in level of consciousness as a haematoma develops which compresses brain tissue and raises ICP. Extradural (between the dura and skull) and subdural (below the dura) haematomas are the most common causes of this complication. Severe secondary brain damage may then occur.

Secondary brain injury is the term given to damage that occurs after the initial trauma as described above. It is frequently caused by cerebral oedema (made worse by high levels of carbon dioxide associated with respiratory difficulties) and raised ICP. This is largely preventable by expert medical and nursing care.

WHAT TO LOOK OUT FOR

Neurological observations (Glasgow Coma Scale) are vital to establish a base-line level of consciousness as soon as the person is admitted to A&E. The first sign of any deterioration will be a reduced level of consciousness, hence frequent repeat neurological observations are essential. The GCS is usually presented in chart form (see Figure 9.2). This may be combined with another chart for further neurological observations and vital signs (see Figure 9.3).

Pupil size and reaction must be monitored (see p665), together with limb movement and power (p691) as follows:

- *Normal power*: limb movements appropriate for the muscle strength of the patient.
- *Mild weakness*: one limb normal, other limb weaker.
- *Severe weakness*: very pronounced difference between the two limbs.
- *Spastic flexion*: slow, stiff movement of the arm with the flexed forearm and hand held against the body.
- *Extension*: elbow or knee joint straightens in response to painful stimulation. This is abnormal as the normal response is flexion away from the painful stimulus.

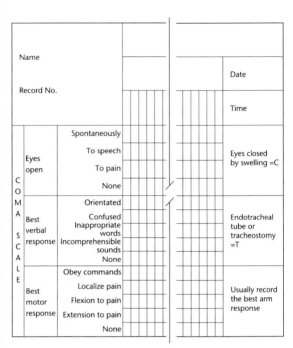

Figure 9.2 Glasgow Coma Scale record sheet.

- *No response*: despite painful stimulation there is no response and the limb remains limp.

A painful stimulus should only be applied by rolling a pencil or biro across the nail bed (see Figure 9.4).

MEDICAL MANAGEMENT

After an initial primary survey upon reception in A&E, the priority is to establish and protect a patent airway whilst immobilizing the cervical spine because of the associated risk of neck injury. High-concentration oxygen via a face mask should be given immediately to reduce the risk of cerebral oedema caused by high carbon dioxide levels. If necessary, the patient will be intubated and ventilated.

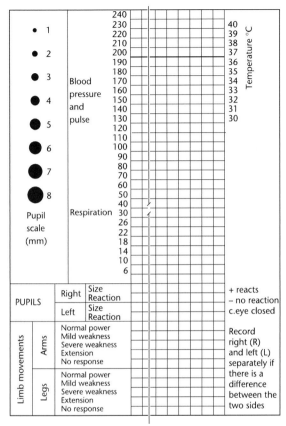

Figure 9.3 Record sheet for other neurological parameters.

If raised ICP is a problem, neurosurgery may be undertaken to deal with the specific problem within the skull (e.g. to drain an epidural haematoma). Further management is directed at reducing cerebral oedema by the use of intravenous osmotic diuretics, such as mannitol and the corticosteroid drug dexamethasone.

The most serious head injuries are usually managed in regional speciality units.

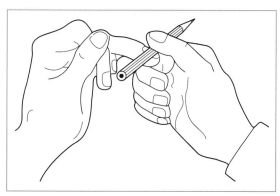

Figure 9.4 Fingernail-bed stimulus.

PHARMACOLOGY FOCUS

Cerebral oedema is one of the main problems in serious head injury. Mannitol is the drug frequently used to tackle this problem. Molecules of the drug are filtered by the glomerulus of the nephron in the kidney, but are not reabsorbed in the tubules. This increases osmolality in the tubules, reduces reabsorption of water, increases urine output and removes fluid from the body. A typical dose is 1 g/kg bodyweight given as a 20% IV solution.

PRIORITIES FOR NURSING CARE

In A&E:

- Frequent, accurate level of consciousness observations using the GCS.
- Assume that a neck injury is present until proven otherwise.
- Close monitoring of vital signs and oxygen saturation.
- Constant monitoring of the patient.
- Immediate availability of suction and oxygen supply.

After admission the above priorities still apply, but in addition:

- Protection of the airway and adequate oxygenation is essential. The patient may be admitted to an intensive care unit for ventilation after intubation in severe injuries.

■ Eye care: periorbital oedema, loss of corneal reflexes and severe bruising around the eyes are often associated with severe head injuries. This requires taping the eye shut to protect the cornea, removing the tape every 2 hours to irrigate the eye with normal saline, instilling artificial tears and then re-taping the eye.

■ If required, maintenance of IV fluid input (and catheter care) combined with accurate fluid balance.

■ Measures to counter hyperthermia should this develop as a result of trauma to the hypothalamus disturbing the temperature-regulating centre.

■ Care of the unconscious patient (if necessary) including key areas such as skin care, nutritional support, mouth care, careful positioning for maximum chest expansion and prevention of limb contractures.

■ Safety precautions should the patient be awake but confused and disoriented.

■ Care of any scalp wound to prevent a potentially serious infection developing.

BRAIN TUMOURS (P711)

PATHOLOGY: Key facts

Tumours may occur at any age and can affect any part of the nervous system, not just the brain. They may be primary, frequently developing from neuroglial tissue (e.g. a glioma). However, the majority are secondary growths (metastases) associated with a distant primary growth elsewhere in the body. Tumours may either be malignant or benign.

As a tumour is a space-occupying lesion, it therefore displaces tissue that would otherwise be there and leads to a rise in intracranial pressure (ICP). Local effects also appear, depending upon which area of the brain is affected. For example, if the pituitary gland is affected endocrine disturbances will follow, while if the cerebrum is involved, behavioural and cognitive abnormalities will result. Some tumours grow very quickly while others grow very slowly making for a great deal of variability in the course of the illness.

WHAT TO LOOK OUT FOR

The patient usually presents initially in primary care. While brain tumours are fortunately relatively rare, the nurse practitioner or practice nurse must be aware of the following warning signs that indicate the need for an immediate medical assessment.

- The onset of symptoms may be gradual with a slow deterioration in mental functioning and/or sensory and motor deficits such as visual disturbances or limb weakness.
- Endocrine disorder may develop if the pituitary is affected.
- Headaches, dizziness, tingling or numbness. However, do remember that headache is a very common symptom and is very unlikely to be associated with a brain tumour.
- Convulsions.
- Other signs and symptoms of raised ICP such as:
  - Deterioration in level of consciousness.
  - Pupillary dysfunction caused by compression of third cranial nerve.
  - Vomiting.
  - Alterations in vital signs. Blood pressure increases, difference between systolic and diastolic BP increases and the pulse slows.
  - Respiratory irregularities.
  - Impaired brainstem reflexes develop in the terminal stages as brain death develops.

MEDICAL MANAGEMENT

Accurate diagnosis of the location and extent of the lesion is made by CT or MRI scanning. Successful surgery offers the best prognosis for the patient. Treatment with the steroid drug dexamethasone will often improve symptoms in the short term by reducing ICP. Tumours that are metastatic in origin, and primary growths such as gliomas, have little response to radiotherapy and chemotherapy. Some other primary tumours do respond, however, to such approaches.

PHARMACOLOGY FOCUS

Dexamethasone is a glucocorticoid drug (steroid), which has a powerful anti-inflammatory effect. Given orally as dexamethasone only, it has an onset time of 1 hour and the effect of a dose lasts up to 3 days. Used to treat raised ICP and cerebral oedema it is given as dexamethasone phosphate which has a very rapid onset of action, quickly reducing oedema and ICP. It is given as an IV injection of 10 mg initially followed by intramuscular injections of 4 mg doses every 6 hours as required up to a maximum of 10 days. Dexamethasone has all the same complications as other steroids.

PRIORITIES FOR NURSING CARE

- Patients will be very anxious as a possible diagnosis of a brain tumour carries with it the fear of death. During the assessment phase, a great deal of support and understanding is needed to help the patient cope with this period of uncertainty. Once the diagnosis is made, further support is needed as required, depending upon the diagnosis and treatment options offered.
- Careful monitoring for signs of rising ICP and other neurological complications will be required during the patient's stay in hospital.
- If surgery is carried out this will be at a specialized centre, which may be some considerable distance from the patient's home, causing difficulties for visiting.
- If the tumour is inoperable, or in the event of recurrence, eventually terminal care will be required. The patient may want to discuss options with the family and health care staff while they are still able. Spiritual care may be especially important at this stage as the patient prepares to face their death.

DEGENERATIVE DISORDERS OF THE NERVOUS SYSTEM (P715)

PATHOLOGY: Key facts

There are a range of degenerative disorders affecting the nervous system for which there is little hope of curative treatment. Four of the principal disorders are summarized below.

Alzheimer's Disease

The most common degenerative brain disorder which often has an onset in middle age. Males and females are equally affected by the widespread loss of nerve cells that occurs, leading to progressive dementia. In the first 2–4 years there is a gradual slow deterioration in mental function which initially may be attributed to forgetfulness and carelessness. Gradually motor function deteriorates, changes in mood such as apathy develop alongside loss of both long- and short-term memory. After a few years it is clear that something is seriously wrong as the patient develops the second stage of the disease. Now they cannot even recognize close friends and relatives (particularly distressing for family members who may have known the person for 40 or 50 years), disorientation is complete and behaviour rambling, disorganized and inappropriate. In the final stages all language is lost, there is total incontinence and the person loses mobility and any kind of meaningful movement, becoming bedridden and helpless.

Multiple Sclerosis

This condition is caused by developing patches of demyelinization affecting neurones in both the brain and spinal cord. Myelin is essential for speedy transit of nerve impulses through axons. Scar tissue replaces the lost areas of myelin, axons degenerate and neurones lose their function. Initially the optic nerves and the spinal cord are most affected. The cause of this condition may lie in a combination of a virus interacting with an autoimmune disorder. Onset is typically in the age range 17–30 years and the incidence of the disease increases in regions where the climate is colder and wetter.

Parkinson's Disease (Paralysis Agitans)

This complex condition is associated with a degeneration of the neurones in the substantia nigra (part of the basal ganglia) and as a result decreased production of the neurotransmitter dopamine. Normal smooth muscle function depends upon a balance between the two neurotransmitters acetylcholine (excitatory) and dopamine (inhibitory) and their actions in the basal ganglia of the brain. In Parkinsonism therefore, there is no dopamine-related function to oppose the action of acetylcholine in the basal ganglia, leading to rigidity throughout the body, tremors and very slow movement. Dopamine depletion so affects muscle function that it also leads to an inexpressive mask-like face, a high-pitched monotone voice, and continual (and very embarrassing) drooling. This disorder can develop under 45 years of age (approximately 10% of patients are under 45 when they first present), but incidence rises steadily with age. Sex incidence is approximately equal.

Motor Neurone Disease

This is characterized by degeneration of motor neurones in the spinal cord and the motor cortex. The disease has a prevalence of 5/100,000 and while some cases do seem to have familial links, the cause of most is unknown. The age of onset is usually over 50 years of age. Presenting symptoms are muscle weakness affecting the limbs and difficulty in swallowing and speech. The disease spreads to affect the whole body with progressive muscle wasting and loss of function leading to total paralysis. Mental function is not normally impaired despite the total paralysis that results.

MEDICAL MANAGEMENT

At present there is little sign of any definitive curative treatment for these diseases although research continues apace and various drug trials are in progress. However, patients with Parkinsonism can be helped by treatment with L-dopa (levodopa), the precursor to dopamine, which replenishes diminished supplies of dopamine in the key areas of the brain where it is needed. Unfortunately some 90% of oral L-dopa is converted to dopamine peripherally and so has no effect on the brain. The drug is usually combined with another drug such as carbidopa which inhibits this peripheral effect and so allows a higher concentration of dopamine to reach the brain.

PRIORITIES FOR NURSING CARE

Patients with these disorders face a steady decline in their ability to function independently. Where cognition remains unaffected, increasing dependence on others is accompanied by the realization that death is approaching. A great deal of support and understanding is therefore required to try and maximize the quality of life that patients may enjoy in the time they have remaining. Spiritual care may be particularly important.

Intensive community care, based around the multidisciplinary team concept, is essential to achieve optimum quality of life for both the patient and family. This may involve short admissions to hospital for respite care and to deal with acute problems as they occur. The primary care nurse therefore plays a major part in supporting these patients.

TEN TOP TIPS

1. Decreasing level of consciousness is the cardinal sign of rising ICP and associated brain pathology.
2. Always assume that any head injured patient has a cervical spine injury until proved otherwise.
3. Maintaining a clear airway and good oxygenation is essential in caring for the unconscious patient.
4. Never forget the importance of pressure area care in looking after patients with any neurological deficit.
5. Remember the importance of limb positioning as contractures develop very quickly and have long-lasting deleterious effects.
6. Avoid giving false hope when patients/families ask about recovery after a CVA.
7. Remember when feeding a patient that swallowing can be seriously impeded after a CVA.

8. Sensory loss can lead to skin lesions which can develop very quickly into serious infected wounds.

9. Always check a confused patient's state of mind before the current presentation, they might have been just as confused before.

10. Avoid using subjective terms like 'semi-conscious' and 'slightly confused'. Use objective measures such as the Glasgow Coma Scale or precise statements such as 'Confused as to time and place'.

Index

Notes: All page references in brackets refer to *Watson's Clinical Nursing and Related Sciences*, 7th edition; page numbers in italics refer to figures and tables.

A

Abortion 130–2
Abscesses 63, 64
Acetylcholine 163
Aciclovir 140
Acidosis 19, 90
Acute heart failure 9
Acute lymphoblastic
    anaemia 45
Acute renal failure (ARF)
    (p621) 120–1
Addison's disease 105
Adenosine triphosphate
    (ATP) 19, 69, 122
Adipose tissue 87
Adrenal cortex 87
Adrenal glands 2, 87, 105
Adrenaline 85, 149
Adrenocorticotropic hormone
    (ACTH) 87, 105
Advanced Breast Biopsy
    Instrumentation
    System 138
Agranulocytosis 102
AIDS (autoimmune deficiency
    disorder) 28, 142
Alanine aminotransferase
    (ALT) 75
Alcohol 62, 74
    abstention 71, 72, 76, 80, 81
    abuse 70, 79
    CAGE screen 73

consumption in UK 72
recommended daily
    intake 73
retention and 116
Aldosterone 8, 87, 111
Alfusozin 117
Alginates 62
Alpha-blocking drugs 117
Aluminium hydroxide 124
Alzheimer's disease 162
Amenorrhoea 134
Amino acids 53, 69, 89, 122
Aminotransferases 70, 75
Ammonia 110
Ammonium 111
Amnesia 154
Amoxicillin 22, 29, 61
Ampulla of Vater 67, 68, 82
Amputation (p850, 852) 12,
    13, 89
Amylase 53, 69, 80
Anaemia (p374) 40–4, 55, 57,
    70, 124, 140
    pernicious 41, 54
    symptoms 42
Anal sphincter 51
Analgesia (p 272) 6
Androgens 116, 119, 134
Aneurysm 152
Anger 153
Angina pectoris (p280) 3–5,
    89, 91
Angiography 12

Angiotensin converting enzyme (ACE) 8, 10
Angiotensin pathway 110
Ankle Brachial Pressure Index 12
Anorexia 47, 48, 63, 70, 92, 134
Antacids 61–2
Anti-emetic drugs 140
Anti-progesterone agent 132
Antibiotics 29, 61, 64, 83
  resistance to 28
Anticholinergic drugs 115
Anticoagulation therapy 14
Antidepressants 116
Antidiarrhoeal agents 64
Antidiuretic hormone (ADH) 86, 105, 111
Antigens 39–40
Antihypertensive drugs 8
Antimicrobial therapy 21, 28, 29, 30, 112, 115
Antimuscarinic drugs 116
Antithyroid drugs 99, 102
Anxiety 5, 11, 23, 92, 102, 153
Aorta 3
Aphasia 153
Aplastic anaemia 41
Appetite 30, 77, 79, 123
Arrhythmias, cardiac 5, 6, 122
Arteriosclerosis 5
Ascites 69, 70, 71, 134
Aspartate aminotransferase (AST) 75
Aspirin 60
Asthma (p338) 23–5, *26*, *27*, 31
Atheroma 3
Atherosclerosis 149
'Atrial systole' 2
Atrioventricular (AV) node 2, *2*
Atrioventricular valves 1
Autocrines 85
Autoimmune disorder 98, 99, 162
Autonomic nervous system 2, 143, 147

Axons (white matter) 146, 148–9, 162
Azathioprine 64

B

Balanitis 91
Barium meal radiography 55, 56, 63
Basal ganglia 145, 163
Basilar artery 146
Bed rest 76, 83
Benign cysts 137
Benign prostatic hyperplasia (BPH) (p774) 116–18, 119
Benign prostatic hypertrophy 115
Benign tumours 159
Benzylpenicillin 29
Berry aneurysm 150
Beta-blockers 8, 10, 102, 149
Beta$_2$-agonists 21, 24–5
Bicarbonate ions 19
Biguanides 94
Bile 59–60, 67, 68–9, 70, 77, 78, 82
Biliary tract *see* Liver, biliary tract and exocrine pancreas
Bilirubin 68, 76, 77
Biopsy 55, 134
  techniques 138
Biphasic insulin 94
Bisoprolol 10
Bladder 135
  anatomy 109
  calculi 112
  function 111, 114, 116, 120, 134
  neck 117
  training programme 115
  wall 113, 115
Bleeding 103, 124, 150
  disorders 77, 79
  vaginal 133
Blindness 89

Blocking agents 8
Blood
  chemistry 32, 121
  composition 36, 38
  count 140
  drainage 1, 3
  groups 39–40
  main functions 38
  osmolarity 110
  pH 19
  red cell formation 35, 44
  tests 56, 70, 75
  values 35, 37
  volume 3, 35, 110
  white cell formation 37,
    44
  see also Glucose levels;
    Haematological system
Blood pressure (BP) 79, 105
  cardiovascular system and 3,
    7, 9–10
  nervous system and 150,
    160
  urinary system and 110,
    123
Blood supply 89
  cardiovascular system and 3,
    5, 13
  nervous system and 149,
    150, 154
  urinary system and 107,
    109
Bone disorders 122
Bone marrow 46, 48
  transplantation 46
Bowel 135
  cancer (p477) 54–5, 56,
    58–9
  disease (p468),
    inflammatory 62–5
Brain 143, 145, 147, 162, 164
  blood supply to 146,
    149–50, 152
  intracranial pressure (ICP)
    and 154–5
  tumours (p711) 159–61
  see also Cerebrum
Brainstem 145–6, 150
  reflexes 160

Breast
  awareness 137
  cancer (p817) 54, 136–41
  implants 138
  screening 137
Breath test 61
Breathlessness 22
British Thoracic Society
    Guidelines 24
Bronchial carcinoma 20
Bronchiectasis 20–1
Bronchodilator drugs 32
Bruising 77, 140
Bundle of His 2, 2
Buserelin 119

C

Calcitonin 87
Calcitrol 110
Calcium 8, 87, 104, 110, 122,
    123
Cancer
  bowel (p477) 54–5, 56, 58–9
  brain tumours (p711)
    159–61
  breast (p817) 54, 136–41
  bronchial carcinoma 20
  of the cervix (p812) 135–6
  of the colon 54
  colorectal 54–5
  gastric 60
  malignant lymphomas
    (p398) 47–9
  metastatic disease 141
  oesophageal (p440) 54, 55,
    56
  ovarian 134
  prostate (p776) 118–20
  stomach (p448) 54, 55, 57–8
  of the thyroid 98
  tumours of the ovary (p811)
    134–5
  see also Cervix (p812),
    carcinoma of the
Carbaminohaemoglobin 19
Carbidopa 164
Carbimazole 99, 102

Carbohydrates 53, 69, 88, 96
Carbon dioxide 18, 19, 31, 38, 90, 155, 156
Cardiac arrhythmias 5, 6, 122
Cardiac sphincter 60
Cardiovascular system 1–15
  anatomy of 1, 2
  angina pectoris (p280) 3–5
  cardiac cycle 1–2
  deep vein thrombosis (DVT) (p319) 13–14, 22, 59, 65, 118
  heart failure (p304) 9–12
  hypertension (p311) 7–9
  myocardial infarction (MI) (p284) 5–7
  peripheral vascular disease (PVD) (p316) 12–13
  physiology of 1–3
  ten top tips 15
Carotid Doppler Ultrasonography 152
Carvedilol 10
Cataract formation 89
Catheters 79, 113, 115, 117–18
Cauda equina 146
Cefotaxime 29
Cellular respiration 19
Central nervous system (CNS) 31, 143, 145–6
Cephalosporins 29, 83
Cerebrospinal fluid (CSF) 146, 154
Cerebrovascular accident (CVA) (p672) 4, 8, 149–54
Cerebrum 145, 159
  cerebral aneurysm 150
  cerebral aqueduct 146
  cerebral artery wall 149
  cerebral contusion 154
  cerebral hypoxia 21, 28, 32, 43
  cerebral ischaemia 154
  cerebral laceration 154
  cerebral oedema 153, 155, 156–7, 158, 161
  cerebral thrombosis 149

Cervix 127
  carcinoma of the (p812) 135–6
Chemotherapy 30, 56, 119, 161
  haematological system and 46–7, 48, 49
  women's health and 134, 138, 139
Chief cells 53
Chlamydia 141
Chloride 110, 111
Chlormethine 48
Cholelithiasis (gallstones) (p517) 70, 78, 82–3
Cholesterol 89, 93
  stones 82
Chronic bronchitis 20, 22
Chronic gastritis 60
Chronic heart failure 9
Chronic hepatitis 70
Chronic kidney disease (CKD) (p610, 615) 9, 120, 122–4
Chronic obstructive pulmonary disease (COPD) (p337) 20–3, 31
Chronic renal failure (CRF) (p615) 89, 122–3
Chyme 59
Cimetadine 61
Circle of Willis 146
Cirrhosis of the liver (p509) 69–73
Clarithromycin 61
Coeliac disease 41
Collecting ducts 108, 109, 110
Colloids 80
Colon 53–4, 63–4
  cancer of 54
Colonoscopy 56, 63
Colostomy 56
Coma 70, 90, 92, 105, 121, 122
Common Bile duct 79, 82
Community care 59, 164
Compression ultrasonography 14
Computed tomography (CT) 55, 152, 160
Concentration 43

Conception, products of 131
Concussion 154
Condoms 76, 113, 116
Confusion 21, 28
  nervous system and 149, 153, 154, 159
  urinary system and 114, 121, 122
Congestive heart failure 9
Consciousness, level of 21, 29
  nervous system and 145, 150–1, 152, 154–5, 160
Constipation 55, 79, 134, 153
Continence 111
Continual ambulatory peritoneal dialysis (CAPD) 123
Contraceptives
  condoms 76, 113, 116
  oral 31, 71
Contrast venography 14
Convulsions 92, 151, 154, 160
Corticosteroids 24–5, 64, 105, 157
Corticotropin-releasing hormone 87
Cortisol 87
Counselling 7
Cranial nerves 143, 147, 160
Creatine phosphokinase (CPK) 6
Creatinine 9, 111, 122
Crohn's disease 41, 62, 63, 64
Cryotherapy 136
Cushing's syndrome 105
Cyanosis 21
Cyclophosphamide 48
Cystadenomas 134
Cystitis 111
Cytokines 46
Cytology 138
Cytotoxic drugs 45, 46, 48

Deep vein thrombosis (DVT) (p319) 13–14, 22, 59, 65, 118
Dehydration 63, 90, 92, 105
Dementia 162
Demyelinization 162
Depolarization, zone of 148
Depression 124, 140, 153
Dermoid cysts 134
Detrusor muscle instability 115
Dexamethasone 157, 160, 161
Diabetes insipidus 105
Diabetes mellitus (p557) 12, 19, 79, 88–98
  classification of 91
  'diabetic coma' 90
  effects on patient 89–90
  insulin injection sites 95
  key diet points 97
  urinary system and 114, 122, 124
Diabetic ketoacidosis 88, 89–90, 92, 93
Diagnostic tests 152
Dialysis 121, 123
Diamorphine 6
Diarrhoea 47, 54, 55, 63, 140
Diastole 1
Diathermy excision 136
Diazepam 71
Diet 44, 58, 96, 121, 124, 153
Digoxin 11
Dihydrotestosterone 117
Disorientation 162
Distal convoluted tubule 108, 109, 111
Distal organ 89
District Nursing 154
Diuretics 8, 10
Dizziness 43, 149
Dopamine 163–4
Doppler ultrasound 12
Doxorubicin 48
Drug addicts 78
Duodenum 68
  duodenal ulcers 59, 60

D

D-Dimer testing 14
Dacron graft 12, 152

Dysphagia 55, 60
Dysplasia 135
Dysuria 112

E

E. coli 112
Electrical conduction system
  2
Electrocardiograph (ECG) 3,
  6, 7
Electroencephalography
  (EEG) 152
Electrolytes 54, 62, 64, 122
  balance of 105, 110, 121,
  123, 124
Embolism 5, 149
  pulmonary 9
Emphysema 20
Endarterectomy 152
Endocrine system 85–106
  anatomy of 85–6, 86
  diabetes mellitus (p557)
  88–98, 91, 95, 97
  disorders 60, 160
  disturbances 159
  function 145
  imbalance in 134
  other disorders
  (p585) 104–5
  physiology of (p551) 86–7
  ten top tips 106
  thyroid disorders (p576)
  98–104, 100–1
Endoscopic retrograde
  cholangiopancreatography
  (ERCP) 82–3
Endoscopy 55, 80
Enterokinase 69
Environmental toxins 74
Epidural haematoma 157
Epinephrine 2, 85, 105, 149
Erythema 140
Erythrocytes (white blood
  cells) 35, 38, 39–40
  production (p375) 37, 40–1,
  44
Erythropoietin 87, 110

Estimated Glomerular
  Filtration Rate
  (eGFR) 122
Exercise 17
  breathing 22
  isometric 7
  plan 4, 11, 98
  tolerance 21, 43
Exocrine pancreas see Liver,
  biliary tract and exocrine
  pancreas
Exophthalmus 99
External beam
  radiotherapy 138
External respiration 18
Eye care 97, 103, 159

F

Faecal impaction 114
Faecal incontinence 153
Faecal occult blood testing 56
Fallopian tubes 127, 133, 134
Family planning advice 132
Family teaching 22–3
Fat tissue 87
Fatigue 5, 48, 63, 74, 77, 92,
  122
Fats 53, 79, 82, 88
  unsaturated 96
Fatty acids 53
Female genitalia 128
Female pelvis 128
Female reproductive
  system 129
Ferrous sulphate 42
Fertility 46, 133
Fetus 129, 131, 132, 133
Fever 63, 77, 82
Fibrosis 95
'Fight or flight response' 147
Filtration 110
Finasteride 117
Fingernail-bed stimulus 156,
  158
Fistula 63, 64
Flatulence 70, 77, 79
Flucloxacillin 29

Fluid balance 83, 102–3, 153, 159
  drinking and 76, 113
  gastrointestinal system and 56, 57, 58, 65
  urinary system and 109–10, 117–18, 121–4
Fluid volume 11
Folic acid 44, 54, 81
  deficiency anaemia 41, 43
Follicle-stimulating hormone (FSH) 129
Furosemide 8

G

Gall bladder 67, *68*, 69
Gallstones (Cholelithiasis) (p517) 70, 78, 82–3
Gangrene 89
Gastrectomy, subtotal 61
Gastric juice 59
Gastric ulceration 54, 60
Gastro-oesophageal reflux disease 62
Gastrointestinal mucosa 140
Gastrointestinal system 51–66
  anatomy of 51–2, *52*
  inflammatory bowel disease (p468) 62–5
  neoplastic disease 54–9
  peptic ulceration (p444) 59–62
  physiology of 52–4
  ten top tips 65–6
Gemeprost 131
Genitalia, female *128*
Glasgow Coma Scale (GCS) 150, *151*, 155
  record sheet *156*
Glibenclamide 94
Gliclazide 94
Gliomas 161
Glomerular filtration rate (GFR) 9, 122
Glomerulus 107, 110, 158
Glucagon 69, 87

Glucocorticoid (steroid) therapy 87, 105, 161
Gluconeogenesis 89
Glucose levels 19, 53, 64, 68–9, 81, 146
  endocrine system and 87, 88, 89, 90, 93, 96
  urinary system and 111, 121, 123
Glucosuria 79, 89
Glycated haemoglobin (HbA$_{1c}$) 93
Glycerol 53
Glycogen 68, 87
Goitre 98
  'toxic goitre' 99
Gonadorelin analogues 119
Goserelin 119
Granulocyte colony stimulating factor 46
Granulocytes 39
Graves disease 99
Grey matter (nucleii) 146
GTN 4, 5
Gum sores 123
Gut 51–2

H

H$_2$-receptor antagonists 61, 62
Haematological system 35–49
  anaemia (p374) 40–4, *42*
  anatomy of 35, *36*, *37*, 38
  leukaemia (p389) 44–7
  malignant lymphomas (p398) 47–9
  physiology of 38–40
  ten top tips 49
Haematoma 139, 154–5
  epidural 157
Haemodialysis 121, 123
Haemoglobin 19, 35, 40, 77
  glycated 93
Haemolytic anaemia (p378) 41
Haemolytic jaundice 77
Haemoptysis 14
Hair loss 47, 140
Hashimoto's disease 98

Head injury (p683) 154–9
Headaches 74, 151, 160
Health education 25, 44
Heart failure (p304) 9–12
Heartburn 60
Helicobacter pylori 54, 59, 61
Hemiplegia 151
Heparin 14
Hepatic coma 70
Hepatitis (p506) 73–6
    chronic 70
    types of viral 74
Hepatocellular jaundice 77
Hepatocytes 73, 77
Heredity, breast cancer
        and 136
Herpes simplex ulcers 140
Hiatus hernia 60
Hirsutism 134
Histamine 60
Hodgkin's disease 47–8
Homeostasis 38
Homosexual patients 76
Hormone replacement
        therapy 99, 102, 137
Hormones 129, 149
Human chorionic
        gonadotrophin 129
Human papillomavirus 135
Hydration 22, 29, 80
Hydrochloric acid 53, 59, 61
Hydrocortisone 24
Hydrogen ions, free 111
Hydroxocobalamin 43
Hyperglycaemia 79, 80, 82, 88,
        89, 105
Hyperglycaemic hyperosmolar
        non-ketotic coma 90
Hypermetabolism 105
Hyperparathyroidism 104
Hyperplasia 20, 116–18, 119
Hypertension (p311) 3, 7–9,
        122, 124, 149
    portal 69
Hyperthermia 159
Hyperthyroidism 98, 99, 102–4
    assessment 100–1
Hypoglycaemia 90, 92, 93, 105
    management of 97

Hypoglycaemics, oral 92, 93,
        94–5
Hypostatic pneumonia 28
Hypotension 105, 117, 120
Hypothalamic-pituitary
        system 105
Hypothalamus gland 85–6,
        86–7, 145, 159
Hypothyroidism 98, 99, 102,
        104
    assessment 100–1
Hypovolaemia 90, 120
Hypovolaemic shock 80
Hypoxia 87
    cerebral 21, 28, 32, 43
Hysterectomy 134, 136

I

Ibuprofen 60
Immunization 75
Immunoglobin 48
Immunosuppressive
        therapy 64
Immunotherapy 46
Incontinence (p633) 113–16,
        162
    extrinsic causes 114
    intrinsic causes 114–15
    physiological causes 113–14
Infection
    abortion and 131
    cervical 135
    chest 22, 32, 118
    control 76
    head injury and 154, 159
    kidney 112
    pelvic 133
    post-chemotherapy 140
    respiratory 122
    urinary tract (UTI) (p641)
        111–13, 114, 115, 116
Inflammatory bowel disease
        (p468) 62–5
Infliximab 64
Inhibitory
        neurotransmitters 149
Injections 94, 95

Insulin 69, 81, 82, 87, 88, 93, 95, 121
Internal respiration 19
International normalized ratio (INR) 14
Interstitial fluid 109–10, 111
Intracranial pressure (ICP) 150–1, 153, 154–5, 157, 159, 160, 161
Intrauterine devices (IUDs) 133
Iodine 98, 102
  radio-iodine treatment 104
Ipratropium 21, 116
Iron 44, 68
Iron deficiency anaemia 40, 42, 43
Islets of Langerhans 60, 79, 85, 87, 88, 94
Isoniazid 30, 74
Itchiness (pruritus) 48, 70, 71, 75, 76, 77, 91, 122

J

Jaundice (p502) 70, 75, 76, 76–8, 82

K

Ketoacidosis, diabetic 88, 89–90, 92, 93
Kidney disease (CKD), chronic (p610, 615) 120, 122–4
Kidneys 8, 87, 89, 90, 107, 109, 158
  cross-section of 108
  donor 123
  infection of 112
Krebs Cycle 19
Kupffer cells 68

L

L-dopa (levodopa) 163
Lactic dehydrogenase (LDH) 6

Lactose 69
Laparoscopy 133
Laparotomy 134
Large intestine 53–4
Large Loop Excision of the Transformational Zone (LLETZ) 136
Laxatives 7
Legislation 130
Lethargy 141
Leucocytes (red blood cells) 30, 38, 44
  formation 30, 38, 44
Leukaemia (p389) 41, 44–7
  acute/chronic 45
Limb, movement and power 151, 155–6, 160
Lipases 53, 69, 78, 80
Lipids 64, 69, 93
Lipoprotein
  cholesterol 93
  low density (LDL) 96
Liver, biliary tract and exocrine pancreas 67–84
  anatomy of 67, 68
  cholelithiasis (gallstones) (p517) 82–3
  cirrhosis of the liver (p509) 69–73
  hepatitis (p506) 73–6, 74
  jaundice (p502) 76–8
  key functions of 68–9
  pancreatitis (p519) 78–82
  physiology of 68–9
  ten top tips 83–4
Liver function tests (LFT) 48, 70
Loop Electrical Excision Procedure (LEEP) 136
Loop of Henle 108, 109, 111
Low-density lipoprotein (LDL) 96
Lucid intervals, head injury and 155
Lumbar puncture 152
Lumpectomy 138

Lungs
  blood supply 13
  disease 9
  see also Respiratory system
Luteinizing hormones (LH)
    119, 129
Lymphatic drainage 139
Lymphocytes 39, 47
Lymphoedema 139
Lymphomas (p398),
    malignant 47–9

M

Magnetic resonance imaging
    (MRI) 48, 152, 160
Malignant lymphomas (p398)
    47–9
Malignant tumours 159
Mammography (Breast X-ray)
    137
Mannitol 157, 158
Marrow hyperplasia 43
Mastectomy 138, 139
Medulla 107
Medulla oblongata 145–6
Megakaryocytes 39
Meglitinides 95
Melaena 75
Memory 162
Menarche, early 136
Meninges 146
Meningitis 154
Menopause 129–30, 136
Menstruation 129, 132
Metabolic acidosis 19
Metastases 119, 135, 138–9,
    141, 159, 161
Metformin 94–5
Metronidazole 64, 83
Microalbuminuria 91
Micturition 111
Midbrain 146
Mifepristone 131, 132
Monoclonal antibodies 46, 64
Monocytes 39
Motor cortex 163
Motor fibres 147

Motor neurone disease 163
Motor skills 153
Mucosa 51, 59
Mucositis 47
Mucus 53, 54, 59
Multidisciplinary team (MDT)
    154, 164
Multiple sclerosis 162
Muscle wasting 163
Muscle weakness 163
Myelin 149, 162
Myocardial infarction (MI)
    (p284) 4, 5–7, 8, 9–10, 89
Myoglobin 6

N

Nateglinide 95
National Health Service (NHS)
    137
Nausea 47, 63, 92, 122, 133,
    140
  liver/pancreas disorders
    and 70, 74, 77, 79, 82
Neck injury 156, 158
Necrosis 120
Needle sharing 76
Neoplastic disease 54–9, 134
  see also Cancer
Nephrons 107, 108, 109, 110,
    111, 158
Nervous system 143–65
  anatomy of (p653) 143–7,
    144
  brain tumours (p711)
    159–61
  cerebrovascular accident
    (CVA) (p672) 149–54
  degenerative disorders
    (p715) 162–4
  head injury (p683) 154–9
  impulse transmission 148–9
  observation chart 155
  physiology of 148–9
  record sheet 157
  ten top tips 164–5
Neuromuscular disease 31
Neuromuscular junction 148

Neurones 143–5, *144*, 148, 162, 163
Neuropathy 88, 89
Neurosurgery 157
Neurotransmitters 148–9, 163
Nifedipine 8
Nipple discharge 137
Nodularity 137
Non-Hodgkin's lymphoma 48
Non-steroidal anti-inflammatory drugs (NSAIDs) 25, 60, 80
Non-sulfonylurea insulin secretagogue 95
Norepinephrine 2, 105
NSAIDs (non-steroidal anti-inflammatory drugs) 25, 60, 80
Nucleii (grey matter) 146
Nulliparous women 136
Nutrition 22, 29, 57, 76
  parenteral 64

O

Obesity 88, 99, 102, 136
Obstructive jaundice 76, 77, 79, 80, 82
Oddi, sphincter of 78
Oedema 10, 70, 121, 134
  cerebral 150, 153, 155, 156–7, 158, 161
Oesophagitis 60
Oesophagus 70
  cancer of (p440) 54, 55, 56–7
  ulceration of 59–60
Oestrogen 116, 129, 138
Oliguria 120
Omeprazole 61
Opiates 71
Opioid analgesia 43, 58, 80
Optic nerves 162
Oral contraceptives 31, 71
Oropharynx 154
Osmolality 158
Ovarian cysts 134

Ovaries 127, 129
  tumours of (p811) 134–5
Ovulation 129
Oxygen 3, 18, 146, 156, 158
  driven nebulizer 24
  levels 31
  saturation levels 21
  supply 43
  therapy 21, 29, 32, 81
  transport 19
Oxyhaemoglobin 19
Oxytocin 86, 131

P

Palliative care 56, 58, 161
  women's health and 134, 138, 141
Pancreas, exocrine *see* Liver, biliary tract and exocrine pancreas
Pancreatitis (p519) 78–82
  acute 78–9, 79, 80, 81
  chronic 79, 80–1, 81–2
Papillomavirus, human 135
Paracentesis 71, 134
Paracetamol 71
Paracrines 85
Paralysis agitans 163
Paralytic ileus 80
Parasympathetic nervous system 2, 147
Parathormone 87
Parathyroid glands 87, 104
  damage to 103–4
Parenteral nutrition 57, 64
Paresis 149
Parietal cells 53, 61
Parkinson's disease 163
Patient teaching 22–3
Patient-controlled analgesia (PCA) 57
Peak expiratory flow rate (PEFR) 23–4, 25
Pelvis, female 114, 115, *128*, 133, 135
Penicillin, antipseudomonal 29
Penis 116

Pepsin 53, 59
Peptic ulceration (p444) 59–62
Percutaneous transluminal coronary angioplasty (PTCA) 4
Peripheral nervous system 143
Peripheral vascular disease (PVD) (p316) 12–13, 89, 91
Peristalsis 109
Peritonitis 61, 79
Pernicious anaemia 41, 54
Phaeochromocytoma 105
Phagocytes 30
Phagocytosis 38, 68
Phosphates 110, 124
Photophobia 151
Physiotherapy 139, 153
Pioglitazone 95
Piperacillin 29
Pituitary gland 85–6, 86–7, 104–5, 145, 159, 160
Plasma 19, 39, 87
Platelets 38, 39
Pneumonia (p334) 25, 28–9
Polarity 148
Pollution, atmospheric 20
Polycystic disease 134
Polyuria 89, 90, 114
Pons Varolii 145
Portal hypertension 69
Post-operative care (p454, 481) 57–8, 58–9, 117–18
Potassium 39, 87, 93
urinary system and 110, 111, 121, 123, 124
Prednisolone 24, 48
Pregnancy (p797) 98, 130–3
ectopic (p796) 133
Pressure areas 22, 43, 152
Primary health care team (PHCT) 23
Procarbazine 48
Prochlorperazine 6
Progesterone 129, 132

Proprioception deficit 153
Prostaglandin 131, 132
Prostate
benign prostatic hyperplasia (BPH) (p774) 116–18, 119, 120
benign prostatic hypertrophy 115
cancer of the (p776) 118–20
obstruction to 112, 114
prostatectomy 117
Prostate specific antigen (PSA) 119
Proteinases 78
Proteins 53, 64, 69, 88, 121
Proteinuria 91
Prothrombin time 70
Proton pump inhibitors 61
Proximal convoluted tubule 108, 109, 111
Pruritus 48, 70, 71, 75, 76, 77, 91, 122
Pseudomucinous cystadenomas 134
Psychological support 7, 21, 23, 47, 49, 56, 65, 81
post-radiotherapy 140
Pulmonary embolism (PE) 9, 13–14
Pulmonary oedema 121
Pulmonary tuberculosis (TB) (p344) 20, 29–31
Pulmonary ventilation 17–18
Pulse oximeter 19
Pupil dysfunction 151, 160
Purkinje fibres 2, 2
Purpura 75
Pyelonephritis 112
Pyloric sphincter 60
Pyrazinamide 30
Pyrexia 47, 48
Pyruvic acid 19

Q

Quadrantectomy 138

R

Radiation 44
Radio-iodine treatment 104
Radioactive implants 138
Radioactive iodine 102
Radiography 48, 49
  skull/spinal 152
Radiology 63
Radiotherapy 55, 56, 119, 139, 161
  haematological system and 46, 47, 48, 49
Ranitidine 61, 81
Reabsorption 111
Reconstructive surgery 138
Rectal digital examination 117
Rectum 63–4, 112
Red blood cells 30, 38, 44
  formation 35, 44
'Releasing' hormones 87
Renal failure
  acute (p621) 120–1
  chronic (CRF) (p615) 89, 122–3
Renal system 108, 110–11
  damage 9
  parenchyma 107
  pyramids 107
Renin 110
Reproductive system, female 129, 136
Respiratory system 17–33
  anatomy of 17, 18
  asthma (p338) 23–5, 26, 27, 31
  chronic obstructive pulmonary disease (COPD) (p337) 20–3, 31
  difficulties 150–1, 155, 160
  infection 122
  obstruction 103
  physiology of 17–19
  pneumonia (p334) 25, 28–9
  pulmonary tuberculosis (TB) (p344) 29–31

respiratory failure (p352) 31–3
  ten top tips 33
Retention of urine 114, 116
Retinae 89
Retinopathy 89
Rifampicin 30–1, 74
Rosiglitazone 95

S

Salbutamol 21, 24, 25, 149
Saline 80
Salpingo-oophorectomy 134
Scar tissue 69, 94, 162
Screening programme (NHS) 137
Scurvy 41
Secondary brain injury 155
Secretion 111
Sensitivity tests 29
Sepsis 31
Serology 61
Seroma 139
Serosa 51
Sexual activity 7, 112, 113, 132, 135
Shock 31, 79, 90, 103, 120, 133
  hypovolaemic 80
Sickle cell disease 41, 43
Sigmoidoscopy 56, 63
'Silent MI' 5
Simmond's disease 105
Sinoatrial (SA) node 2–3, 2
Skin
  breakdown 89, 140
  care 76, 97, 102, 103, 124, 159
Skull see Head injury
Slurred speech 149
Small intestine 53
Smoking 60, 62, 98, 135
  cardiovascular system and 4, 7, 8, 11, 12, 13
  respiratory system and 20, 21, 22
Social isolation 153

Sodium 8, 39, 87, 110, 111, 121, 148
Somatic nervous system 143
Speech 163
  disturbance (aphasia) 153
Sperm banking 49
Spider angiomas 70
Spinal cord 114, 143, 146, 147, 162, 163
Spinal nerves 143, 147
Spiritual care 161, 164
Spironolactone 8
Spontaneous abortion 130
Squamocolumnar junction (cervix) 135
Staphylococcus 29
Steatorrhoea 79, 81
Stem cell transplantation 46
Sterility 134
Steroid therapy 64, 160, 161
Stomach 53
  cancer (p448) 54, 55, 57–8
  ulceration 59
Stool cultures 63
Stress 60, 102, 147
Stress incontinence 114, 115
Subarachnoid haemorrhage 150
Submucosa 51
Substantia nigra 163
Sulfasalazine 64
Sulphonylureas 94–5
Suppurative pneumonia 20
Surgery
  brain tumours 160, 161
  breast cancer 138
  bypass 12, 55
  Crohn's disease 64
  ectopic pregnancy 133
  gastrointestinal system (p454, 481) 57–8, 58–9
  hysterectomy 136
  oesophageal cancer 55–6
  ovarian tumours 134–5
  pancreatitis 80
  peptic ulceration 61
  prostate 115, 117–18, 119
  reconstructive 138
  subtotal thyroidectomy 99, 103
  therapeutic abortion 131
  transient ischaemic attacks (TIA) and 152
Swallowing 163
Sweating 92
Sympathetic nervous system 2, 8, 147
Synapse 148–9
Systole 2

T

Tachycardia 92, 120
Tamoxifen 138–9
Tattoos 76
Teflon graft 12
Terbutaline 21
Terminations see Abortion
Testosterone 117
Tetany 104
Thalami 145
Thalassaemia 42
Therapeutic abortion 130, 131, 132
Thiamine 54
Thiazolidinediones 95
Thromboemboli 135
Thrombosis 149
  therapy (p287) 6
Thrombus 5
Thyroid gland 87
  disorders (p576) 98–104, 100–1
Thyroid-stimulating hormone (TSH) 87
Thyroidectomy, subtotal 99
Thyrotoxicosis 104
Thyrotrophin-releasing hormone 87
Tolterodine 115
'Toxic goitre' 99
Tranquillizers 116
Transient ischaemic attacks (TIA) 149, 152

Transplants
    heart 10
    liver 71
Transurethral resection of the
    prostate (TURP) 117
Trauma 31, 159
Tremors 92
Triglycerides 68, 69, 87, 93
Trimethoprim 112
'Triple therapy' 61
Tripsinogen 69
Troponin 6
Tru-cut technique 138
Trypsin 53
Tuberculosis (TB) (p344),
    pulmonary 29–31
Tumours
    brain (p711) 159–61
    ovarian (p811) 134–5
    pituitary 105

U

Ulceration
    gastric 54, 60
    of oesophagus 59–60
    oral mucosa 43
    peptic (p444) 59–62
Ulcerative colitis 62, 63
Ultrasound 12, 80, 133, 137
Uraemia 120, 124
Urea 110, 111
Ureters 109
Urethra 109, 111, 112
Urge incontinence 115
Urinary system 107–25
    anatomy of 107–9, 108
    benign prostatic hyperplasia
        (BPH) (p774) 116–18,
        119, 120
    chronic kidney disease
        (CKD) (p610, 615) 9,
        120, 122–4
    drainage 117
    incontinence (p633) 113–16
    physiology of 109–11
    prostate cancer (p776)
        118–20

renal failure (p621, 615)
    120–1, 122–4
    retention 114, 116
    ten top tips 125
    testing 9, 77, 91, 93, 112,
        113, 114–15
Urinary tract infection (UTI)
    (p641) 111–13, 114, 115,
    116
Uterus 127, 129, 131, 133, 134,
    136
    contractions of 132

V

Vagina 112, 127, 131, 133, 135
Vagotomy 61
Vagus nerve 61, 147
Vascular occlusion 43
Vasopressin 86
Venous drainage 3
Ventilation, pulmonary 17–18
Ventricles 146
Vincristine 48
Vision 149, 151, 153, 160
Vital signs 150, 152, 155, 158,
    160
Vitamins 124
    A 68, 81
    B$_{12}$ 41, 43, 44, 58, 68, 81
    C 41, 44
    D 68–9, 81, 110, 123
    E 68
    K 54, 68, 79, 81
Voluntary nervous system 143
Vomiting 47, 74, 77, 79, 82, 92
    nervous system and 151,
        160
    women's health and 133, 140
Vulva 127, 128

W

Warfarin 14, 31
Weight loss 48, 70, 77, 79
    cardiovascular system and 4,
        8, 11

Weight loss (*contd*)
  chemotherapy and 47
  endocrine system and 98,
    99, 103
  respiratory system and 22,
    30
White blood cells 35, 38,
  39–40
  production (p375) *37*, 40–1,
    44
White matter (axons) 146
Women's health 127–42
  abortion and 130–2
  anatomy and 127, *128*
  breast cancer and (p817)
    136–41
  carcinoma of the cervix and
    (p812) 135–6
  physiology and 129–30
  pregnancy and (p797, 796)
    130–3
  ten top tips 141–2
  tumours of the ovary (p811)
    and 134–5
World Health Organization
  (WHO) 30

Z

Zollinger-Ellison syndrome
  60